Exercising Your Way to Better Mental Health

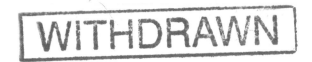
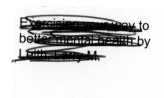

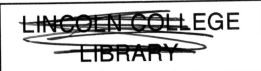

Exercising Your Way to Better Mental Health

Combat stress, fight depression, and improve your overall mood and self-concept with these simple exercises

Larry M. Leith

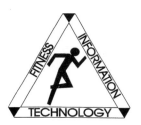

Fitness Information Technology, Inc.

P.O. Box 4425, University Avenue
Morgantown, WV 26504-4425 USA

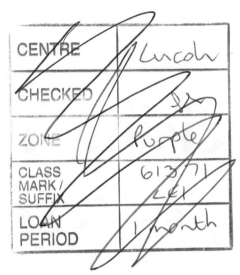
Copyright © 1998 by Larry M. Leith

Photograph credits: Cover photograph by The Stock Market
Photos within each chapter are by the author.

Library of Congress Card Catalog Number: 97-61333

ISBN 1-885693-09-5

Cover Design: Lightbourne Images
Copyeditor: Sandra R. Woods
Proofreader: Maria denBoer
Production Editor: Craig Hines
Printed by: BookCrafters

Printed in the United States of America
10   9   8   7   6   5   4   3

Fitness Information Technology, Inc.
P.O. Box 4425, University Ave.
Morgantown, WV 26504-4425 USA
(800) 477–4348
(304) 599–3482 (phone/fax)
E-mail: fit@fitinfotech.com
Website: www.fitinfotech.com

NOTICE

The exercises, psychological interventions, and assessments referred to in this book should be performed by individuals with appropriate training. The exercises prescribed are not intended for use by the general public without appropriate evaluation and supervision by physicians and certified exercise specialists. This book is not intended to suggest that exercise can replace medication in those individuals who require it. Further, because people respond differently to various exercise programs, it cannot be guaranteed that the exercises advocated in this book will always result in improvements in mental health. Finally, all individuals portrayed in the case anecdotes are fictitious characters — any resemblance to living persons is purely coincidental.

ABOUT THE AUTHOR

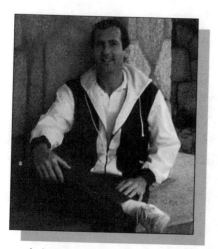 Dr. Larry M. Leith is a professor in the School of Physical and Health Education at the University of Toronto. He holds a cross appointment with the Department of Behavioral Sciences in the Faculty of Medicine. Larry teaches undergraduate courses in sport psychology and health psychology, as well as a graduate course in exercise psychology. Larry has presented and published over one hundred articles dealing with health psychology, sport psychology, and other areas of human behavior. He enjoys taking part in physical activity even more than writing about it. His favorite exercises are walking and jogging, while tennis and golf represent his favorite sports. Larry and his wife Nancy reside in Guelph, Ontario.

CONTENTS

ACKNOWLEDGMENTS

There are many people to thank for their contribution during the writing of this book. First, my wife and best friend Nancy — thanks for your encouragement, understanding, and helpful suggestions. The book also benefited greatly from the reviews of Dr. Frank Perna, Ms. Nita Wood, and Mr. Phil Ancheril. All three of these individuals spent many hours reviewing the work and offering advice to make the book as comprehensive and user-friendly as possible. Similarly, the copyeditor, Sandra Woods, contributed significantly to the quality of this work. I am also grateful to the exercisers who graciously allowed me to use their photographs throughout the book. Finally, my sincere thanks to Dr. Andrew Ostrow, President, Fitness Information Technology, Inc., for his constant support, feedback, and thorough understanding of the publication process.

PREFACE

In 1994, my previous book, *Foundations of Exercise and Mental Health*,[1] was published. It represented the most thorough and comprehensive review of the exercise and mental health relationship available on the market. In preparing that book, I reviewed over 700 published studies, including over 250 research experiments. All of this information was used to provide specific exercise prescription guidelines. Soon after its publication, I received numerous requests to appear on national TV news and talk shows and to give community talks on this important subject. In almost every instance, I was asked the same question: "Wouldn't it be great if this information was available to the general public?" After several discussions with my publisher, Andrew Ostrow, President, Fitness Information Technology, we decided to publish a book that was more appropriate for the general public and that could be made available in local bookstores.

Exercising Your Way to Better Mental Health is based on the research reported in my previous book. It provides a series of checklists and worksheets to increase your self-awareness, and gives specific exercise guidelines to help you improve your mental health. This latest book is intended for those individuals who are having troubles with low self-concept, depression, and stress/anxiety. However, it will be of equal interest to the reader who is not experiencing mood problems, but wishes to improve his or her overall level of wellness.

In chapter 1, you are introduced to the prevalence of mental health problems, and learn how exercise has the potential to improve your overall mental health.

Chapters 2, 3, and 4 look specifically at the issues of self-concept, depression, and stress/anxiety. Each of these chapters provides the tools to recognize the problem, then tells you how to use exercise to improve your mood. You also learn what exercises work best, as well as how often, how hard, and how long you must exercise to get the beneficial results.

Chapter 5 then exposes you to six different types of exercise that have been shown to improve mental health. It provides all of the information you need to choose an activity, including the advantages of that exercise, required equipment, proper technique, and some final helpful hints. This chapter also presents sample exercise programs for beginners to help get you started.

Chapter 6 exposes you to a series of behavioral tools that will help you stick with your exercise program. All of the techniques presented in this chapter have been found to be effective in exercise maintenance.

Finally, chapter 7 provides you with a personal exercise diary. In this diary, you are encouraged to record your weekly exercise sessions and specific moods. This way, you can see your progress firsthand.

In conclusion, it is gratifying to write a book that has so much potential to improve the reader's quality of life. I hope that you will put the principles in this book to work for you. If you do, you will soon learn the value of exercise in promoting positive mental health.

Note

1. Leith, L.M. (1994). *Foundations of exercise and mental health.* Morgantown, WV: Fitness Information Technology, Inc.

Chapter 1

Introduction

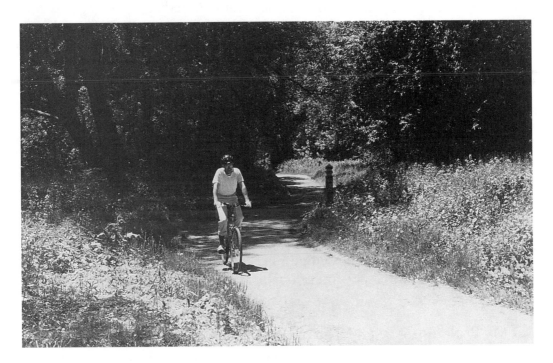

If you think you could use a little boost with your mood from time to time, then rest assured: you are not alone. In this fast-paced, stressful world, it is natural to experience day-to-day mood swings. Sometimes, they are minor

---

In this chapter, we will

✓ outline the prevalence of mental health problems.

✓ explain how exercise can improve mental health.

✓ put your mind at ease about the exercise process.

✓ show how it isn't necessary to become a fitness fanatic to enjoy the mental health benefits of regular exercise.

✓ indicate how to use this book most effectively.

---

inconveniences. Other times, however, they can be a cause for serious concern. In either case, this book should be of considerable value.

For example, you might be interested to know that in any six-month span, 20% of the adult population experiences some form of mental disturbance. This represents approximately 40 million individuals in North America alone. In addition, it has been estimated that almost four out of every 10 people experience a significant psychiatric problem at some point in their lifetimes. This statistic represents almost 80 million North Americans. Add to this the fact that only one out of every five of these individuals will seek medical help, and you will start to realize the scope of the problem.

As a final point of interest, almost one-half of all visits to medical practitioners are termed "stress-related." I'm sure you know that the traditional form of treatment for these kinds of problems involves the use of some form of medication, or pills. While this approach can often improve the disorder, it can also involve some serious side effects. For example, many popular traditional medications are accompanied by side effects such as dry mouth, nausea, constipation or diarrhea, blurred vision, dizziness, headache, disturbed sleep patterns, and even fainting. In addition, taking some medications for a prolonged period of time can result in addiction. Coming off this type of medication almost always results in symptoms of withdrawal. Withdrawal typically involves a set of flu-like symptoms, such as nausea, dizziness, fatigue, and restlessness. Fortunately, the side effects of some newer drugs are not as severe or frequent.

But My Problems Are Not That Severe

While not everyone experiences mood problems serious enough to require medical help, almost all of us do have our ups and downs from time to time. The concepts we will cover in this book will prove beneficial even if you have never considered going to a doctor for help. This is because the principles of mood exercise have the potential to work just as well for minor problems as they do for major ones. **Even better, if you exercise on a regular basis, the chances are good that you will actually be able to prevent a variety of mood disturbances, such as depression, anxiety, low self-esteem, anger, and even mental fatigue.**

In summary, the exercises provided in this book can help you in three different ways. First, they can help prevent mood problems from occurring. Second, they can significantly improve a variety of mood disorders that you experience on a day-to-day basis. Third, even if the problems are severe enough for you to seek medical help, exercise can provide a valuable boost to the more traditional treatments prescribed by your doctor.

Brenda's Blahs

For about six weeks, Brenda's mood seemed to be gradually deteriorating. She felt depressed and stressed out for no apparent reason, and had trouble sleeping. Although she didn't feel that her problems were serious enough to see a doctor, she did notice they were affecting the way she felt during most of the day. These feelings were made worse by her lack of sleep. Brenda considered trying some of the over-the-counter sleeping tablets, but didn't really feel comfortable with this idea either. One day, during a conversation with a close friend, she was told about a book that outlined a program of exercise to improve mood. Although this seemed like a somewhat different idea, she decided to give it a try. In no time, Brenda was glad she did. She noticed improvements with the first exercise session, but better yet, these feelings continued to improve over her first several weeks of exercise. She still feels down from time to time, but overall her mood has been greatly improved by this simple program.

The Traditional View of Exercise

Most people already have a fair idea about the physical benefits of exercise for their bodies. Exercise physiologists have documented several important bodily changes that accompany participation in an ongoing exercise program. Let's take a moment to summarize several of these key physical improvements, which include:

- decreased chance of heart disease and stroke
- increase in good (HDL) cholesterol
- decrease in bad (LDL) cholesterol
- lowered risk of osteoporosis ("brittle bones")
- decreased percentage of body fat
- increased lean muscle mass
- lower blood pressure
- improved immune system

How Can Exercise Improve Mental Health?

One of the questions I am most frequently asked when giving talks on this subject is, "How can exercise possibly improve a person's mental health?" Most people usually go on to say they understand how exercise improves the body, but these same individuals find it hard to believe that exercise can also improve the mind. This is certainly understandable and probably stems from people's traditional view of exercise.

Recent evidence, however, helps shed some light on this difficult question. At this time, there is no one correct answer. Several theories attempt to explain the relationship between exercise and mental health.

The most popular explanation suggests that during exercise, the brain releases *endorphins*. These naturally occurring body chemicals are similar to morphine. For this reason, endorphins have also been called "feel-good" chemicals and have been found to be particularly important in regulating emotion and perceiving pain. According to this viewpoint, when a person exercises, the brain releases endorphins into the bloodstream. These endorphins then cause the individual to feel better emotionally, or put another way, they improve his or her mood. Although this explanation remains popular, the endorphin theory has not been scientifically verified.

A second popular argument is called the *monoamine hypothesis*. This argument suggests that low- to moderate-intensity exercise, by placing the body in a *good stress response* situation, causes the release of brain chemicals called monoamines. These, in turn, are believed to be responsible for making us feel better. Most readers can more easily relate to the effect of these chemicals on the body from a *bad stress response*. For example, if you are walking along a sidewalk and a large dog comes running out, barking and showing its teeth, your fright or fear feeling is largely due to the release of monoamines. Similarly, if you are attempting to catch a bus and it pulls away from the bus stop just seconds before you arrive, that surge of energy you experience as you run the last little distance is also the result of monoamines. In both of these cases, you will readily admit that the feeling is not nearly so pleasant.

Of special interest to the reader is the finding that the number and amount of these chemicals available along the neural pathways of the brain are related to our moods. If insufficient amounts of these monoamines are available in a person's brain, then mood disorders, such as depression and anxiety, are more likely to occur. From this finding, it seems logical to assume that if exercise increases the amount of brain monoamines, it will, therefore, improve mood. This argument makes even more sense when you consider that drug companies produce medications, such as antidepressants, that have the primary function of improving the balance of these brain chemicals. Exercise may indeed accomplish this naturally.

A third explanation of how exercise can improve our mood is called the *thermogenic hypothesis*. People supporting this position point out how exercise results in body warming. Anyone who has ever attempted to exercise will appreciate that exercise does indeed result in body warming — that's why we sweat. This idea is by no means a new one. The therapeutic effect of elevating body temperature has been recognized for several hundred years. Scandanavians regularly take sauna baths for both health benefits and the feeling of well-being. This practice appears to make sense because research has shown that whole-body warming, such as a warm bath or sauna bathing, results in reduced muscle tension. Perhaps this is why so many individuals like to enjoy a long, hot shower or a warm bath to unwind after a difficult day. Exercise, then, does much the same thing. It results in body warming, caused by the release of pyrogens into the bloodstream. This body warming then relaxes our muscles and makes us feel better.

So far, all of these explanations can be termed biochemical in origin. But it appears there may be psychological reasons as well as biochemical ones for the effect of exercise on mood.

An alternative explanation is called the *distraction theory*. This viewpoint maintains that exercise can provide a form of time-out from whatever is bothering us. In this way, exercise can take our minds off depressing or anxiety-producing thoughts. By giving us something else to do and think about, exercise removes us, at least temporarily, from our day-to-day problems. When this feature is combined with the biochemical effects of exercise, the overall result is to improve the participant's mood.

A final explanation for the way exercise can improve our moods is the *self-efficacy theory*. In its simplest terms, self-efficacy is really only a form of confidence in completing a specific task. This viewpoint predicts that engaging in a workout will make us feel better about ourselves, simply because we have done something worthwhile. Frequent comments you have heard in a locker room (or maybe even said yourself), such as, "At least I have accomplished something today," will help you relate to this explanation. After a workout, we feel good about ourselves because we have done something worthwhile. This boost to self-confidence then carries over into other aspects of our mood.

In summary, several theories have attempted to explain how exercise can improve our moods. Many researchers now believe that the monoamine, thermogenic, and self-efficacy theories have the most merit. However, no single explanation has proved superior. Perhaps the most logical conclusion is that several of these processes may occur at once, possibly combining their effects to produce the improved mood benefits. But then again, you are probably much more interested in the fact that exercise does indeed improve your mood rather than being able to explain the reason why. Let's leave that to the experts, and simply enjoy the fact that exercise makes us feel better both physically and mentally.

What If I Don't Know Much about Exercise?

If you have not had much experience with exercise, or don't know much about it, don't worry. This book will walk you through all the steps you need to know to start using exercise to improve your mood.

Chapter 5 will present all the information you need to determine a suitable exercise program that will meet your needs. We will go over different types of exercises that have been shown to improve mental health and tell you how often, how hard, and how long you should exercise to experience mental health benefits. We will also provide sample beginning programs for each type of exercise.

Other chapters will then apply these principles to help you determine the best exercise program to improve self-concept and reduce depression and anxiety. In addition, a separate chapter will outline proven techniques that will help you stick to your program.

As a final aid, the last chapter will provide you with a personal exercise diary. In this diary, you can record your daily and weekly exercise, as well as comments on how you feel both before and after the exercise sessions.

But Is Exercise Safe?

Before starting your actual exercise program, you should determine with certainty that exercise poses no health risk. At the beginning of chapter 5, we will take you through an established procedure to help you answer this question. You will be asked to complete a Personal Health Checklist as a screening step. The way you answer these questions will tell you whether or not you need to check with your doctor before starting an exercise program. So if you are worrying about whether or not exercise is safe, rest assured that you will be given all the help you need to answer this important question.

Do I Have to Become a Fitness Fanatic?

You will probably be pleased with this answer. To experience the benefits of improved mental health from exercise, you need not spend a great deal of time exercising. When most people think about an exercise program, they conjure up visions of sweating and labored breathing throughout a workout. But remember, we are talking about mental fitness here, not physical fitness. This is an important distinction. In several of the later chapters, you will read how fitness gains are not necessary for you to improve your overall self-concept, fight depression, and combat stress. In fact, it is not even necessary to engage in vigorous workouts to experience the desired benefits. As long as you do the appropriate exercises for the correct length of time, you will enjoy the mental health benefits, even if you work out at a mild level of intensity.

This book will provide you with all of the information you need to get started on the road to better mental health.

How to Use This Book

Take a few minutes and read through the following section. It will tell you how to use this book in the most effective way.

Step 1

Make the commitment to improve your mental health with exercise. If you are currently having problems with depression, high stress, anxiety, or poor self-concept, then the principles outlined in this book should prove helpful over the next few weeks. In addition, even if you are not experiencing any of the above problems, this book can still be of value. Recent research has shown that exercise may be just as effective in preventing mental health problems as it is in treating them. So either way, by following the simple exercise program suggestions provided in this book, your overall mental health is going to benefit.

Step 2

This step is one of the most important. If you feel you could use the information provided in this book, it is absolutely essential that you determine if exercise is safe for you as an individual. As mentioned earlier, you will be provided with all of the tools to answer this question at the beginning of chapter 5. So before you proceed any further, turn to that section of the book and honestly answer the simple questions in the Personal Health Checklist.

Step 3

If you are currently experiencing problems with depression, high stress, anxiety, or poor self-concept, then simply turn to the appropriate chapter in this book to find out how to use exercise to combat the problem. Each of these chapters will provide valuable background information on the problem area, then outline specific exercises that have been highly effective in bringing about improvements. You will also learn how often, how hard, and how long you need to perform these exercises to bring about the desired changes. Finally, you will be provided with a guideline in terms of how long it will be before you notice improvements.

If you wish to begin an exercise program to prevent problems or to improve your overall mental health in the absence of problems, then this book will be effective in this regard. You may want to read through the book cover to cover to become more informed about the areas where you will notice improvement.

Step 4

Regardless of the reason you choose to exercise, your next goal is to read through the remainder of chapter 5. This will provide you with all of the information you need to select an exercise that has the most appeal to you.

Step 5

Before you start your exercise program, make sure you take advantage of all of the information provided in chapter 6. This will help you stick with your exercise program. All of the principles discussed have been developed from research on behavior-change strategies. Following these guidelines will greatly improve your chances of becoming a regular exerciser, thereby improving your mental health.

Step 6

Use the personal exercise diary in chapter 7 to keep track of your physical activity, daily mood, and any other information that is important to you. This diary will help you see patterns and provide a record of your progress toward improved mental health.

Looking Back

In this chapter, you have seen that problems with mood are by no means your private domain. A large number of the adult population experience problems with poor self-concept, depression, stress, and anxiety. Traditionally, people seek medical advice and often wind up taking a variety of medications. While this approach is warranted in certain circumstances, it is not always the answer. For the many individuals who do not require medical help, and even for those who do, exercise has been shown to be a valuable treatment option. In addition to providing a wide range of physical benefits, exercise has now been shown to have great potential to improve mental health. Several explanations were provided to help you understand this relationship, and it is probably some combination of all of them that makes exercise work. Even if you don't know much about exercise, this book will provide all of the information you need to start experiencing the positive mood benefits associated with regular participation in physical activity.

CHAPTER 2

IMPROVING YOUR SELF-CONCEPT WITH EXERCISE

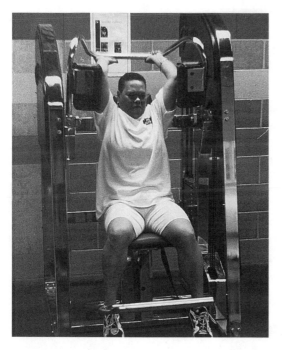

All of us have self-doubts at one time or another. This is only natural as we deal with new situations in the course of daily living. Starting a new job, project, or relationship is often associated with apprehension as we struggle to convince ourselves that we are up to the task. How often or how severely we experience this self-doubt is related to our overall level of self-concept. The better our self-concept, the less we tend to doubt our abilities. The worse our self-concept, the more we seriously question our potential to perform successfully. When this happens, we tend to avoid situations

In this chapter, we will
- ✓ talk about the meaning of self-concept.
- ✓ consider just how important self-concept really is.
- ✓ learn to recognize problems with self-concept.
- ✓ look at how doctors traditionally treat these problems.
- ✓ explore how exercise can improve the way we feel about ourselves.
- ✓ look at what exercises are best to improve self-concept.
- ✓ learn how hard, how long, and how often we must exercise to obtain the desired benefits.
- ✓ suggest a time frame for noticing improvements.

where we feel failure is inevitable. Obviously, this is no way to lead our lives. For this reason, it is important to explore ways we can improve our overall self-concept in an attempt to have a more enjoyable and rewarding life.

After reading this chapter, you will have a tailor-made, inexpensive approach to improving your self-concept. Better yet, you can determine your own schedule for self-help.

Tom's Termination

Tom had been a devoted, hard-working employee of the company for over 10 years before the axe fell. Downsizing was the only explanation given when he received his pink slip. Although the first few weeks of unemployment were a bit of a treat, it didn't take long for the novelty to wear off. Within a short time, Tom's self-confidence was at an all-time low. Although his wife tried to cheer him up, there was only so much she could do. She became worried, however, when she noticed that he started drinking more, and even took up smoking again — something he had quit years before. About the same time, Tom lost interest in socializing with their regular friends. He started gaining weight and became irritable with his wife and children. She suggested that Tom seek the help of a counselor. Although Tom benefited from having someone to talk to, he still didn't feel as if he were making the necessary progress. He took the advice of his counselor and started an exercise program. It wasn't easy to try a new activity, but after the first few weeks, Tom began to feel better about himself. He lost the weight he had gained, quit smoking, and felt comfortable seeing his old friends. As Tom put it, "It was a great feeling to take charge of my own life again, and know that I was actually doing something to make the problem go away." Armed with this new attitude, Tom was soon out looking for work.

What Exactly Is Self-Concept?

Although academics have a wide range of definitions, self-concept is basically a form of trust and belief in our own abilities. Trust and belief in ourselves develop from our sum total of personal experiences, past behaviors, and social interactions. Whether we know it or not, we are continually comparing ourselves with others to see how we measure up. When all of these conscious and unconscious comparisons are added up in our minds, they result in the development of our self-concept. This in turn tends to predict how we will evaluate our chances of success in upcoming events.

Our overall self-concept probably develops from a large number of more specific self-concepts. In other words, all of us have a variety of aspects to our lives, such as physical prowess, social skills, emotional makeup, and strength of intellect. Obviously, we will be stronger in some of these dimensions than in others. In fact, we may be quite poor in any one of these categories, but this does not mean that we will necessarily have a low self-concept. This is because our mind tends to process our relative abilities in all of these skills, then comes up with an overall evaluation by summing the parts. This is an important point. Later in this chapter you will see how exercise has the potential to improve your mental health by restructuring how you view yourself in one or more particular dimensions.

Finally, it is important to distinguish between self-concept and self-esteem. Although these words are often used interchangeably, they actually mean two different things. You have already seen that self-concept refers to our overall analysis of ourselves along a variety of dimensions.

Self-esteem, on the other hand, adds a more emotional component to the evaluation. Perhaps the best definition of self-esteem is "the degree to which individuals feel positive about themselves." When seen in this light, self-esteem is a personal judgment of worthiness. Because it is almost impossible to consider a picture of ourselves without experiencing some degree of self-evaluation, it is probably okay to use the terms *self-concept* and *self-esteem* interchangeably. Remember, though, that self-esteem is more closely linked to emotion or how you feel about yourself, while self-concept is more closely linked to various comparisons of your relative abilities.

Why Is Self-Concept So Important?

Most experts believe that self-concept is the best indicator of overall emotional adjustment. Over the years, some excellent scholars have shown that underlying feelings of worthlessness usually go hand in hand with mental illness. For this reason, most types of client-centered therapy have as a primary goal the improvement of self-concept and self-esteem.

A fairly substantial body of research has shown that self-esteem is inversely related to anxiety in the general population. In other words, the lower the self-esteem, the greater the likelihood that that person is experiencing problems with stress and anxiety. Similarly, acute levels of depression have also been consistently associated with lower self-esteem. And finally, low self-esteem has also been linked to problems of neurosis, child abuse, substance abuse, and poor adolescent interpersonal relations.

When we consider all of the previously discussed facts, it becomes obvious that the development of a positive self-concept is a critical goal. In this chapter, you will see how exercise has great potential not only to make you feel better about yourself, but also to help prevent a variety of other associated problems.

How Can I Recognize Problems with Self-Concept?

It is usually relatively easy to recognize people who are suffering from low self-concept. These individuals frequently employ self-deprecatory state-ments and run themselves down for no apparent reason. In addition, they tend to demonstrate several other consistent patterns. If you are interested in seeing how you stack up against these symptoms, read through the following checklist and mark those items that apply to you on a regular basis.

LOW SELF-CONCEPT CHECKLIST

Feelings of worthlessness _____

Tendency to avoid groups _____

Unwillingness to try new activities _____

Feelings of failure _____

Avoidance of eye contact with others _____

Poor posture _____

Since all of us experience some of these symptoms from time to time, there is no need to worry unless you are experiencing several on a regular basis. If this applies to you, read through this chapter and see how you can start making noticeable progress toward a more positive self-concept.

How Is Low Self-Concept Usually Treated?

The specific treatments for low self-concept are usually determined by the background orientation of the therapist. In other words, the caregiver uses the technique with which he or she is most familiar. Even so, two particular treat-ments appear especially helpful in dealing with problems of low self-concept.

Group therapy is one technique that has proven to be effective in bring-ing about positive change. With this type of therapy, the group serves as a testing ground in which clients suffering from low self-concept try new behaviors and test new ideas. Group members provide feedback to the indi-vidual and often suggest different ways of responding. This approach is believed effective in promoting self-esteem because everyone in the group can occasionally provide help for another member. The group is also a set-ting in which genuine concern can be expressed. Once more adaptive behav-iors are learned, the group helps the individual maintain these new behav-iors. The best results usually occur when the group is made up of members who have similar types of problems, such as obesity or substance abuse. A final advantage of group therapy is that it often provides an opportunity for the development of new friendships formed within the group. This in itself can result in more positive feelings.

A second effective treatment for low self-concept is *cognitive therapy*, which involves the use of self-talk and visual imagery to help guide behavior. The client and therapist develop a series of positive statements or images designed to improve self-concept. The client then practices these self-statements and visual images until they become second nature.

For example, people wishing to improve their self-concept would learn to prompt themselves with statements such as, "I'm just as good as the next person," or, "Today, I'm going to feel really good about myself." An even stronger self-statement, such as "I am a worthwhile individual with a lot to offer," could be repeated throughout the day. Since there is evidence that how we think determines how we feel, this technique should result in improved self-concept.

As a somewhat different approach, several therapists teach their clients to use positive *visual imagery* to improve the way they feel about themselves. The use of imagery can best be explained by the phrase "seeing a picture through your mind's eye." For example, a person could practice seeing a mental picture of himself or herself walking confidently down the street, feeling wonderful. Or more specifically, the individual may think of a problem situation, such as talking with a parent, then develop a "mental movie" of this situation in which the outcome turns out favorably.

This technique has been even more effective if the user learns to experience the good feeling that goes along with such a positive outcome. In summary, the main idea is that these positive self-statements and positive imagery become a natural way of thinking. When this happens, they will invariably improve the person's self-concept. But to be effective, these techniques must be practiced regularly. There is also a tendency for the client to slip back into his or her old way of thinking once away from the influence of the therapist. For this reason, it would prove helpful if there was a different form of self-maintenance that could provide us with the same results.

In the remainder of this chapter, you will see how exercise can perform this important function.

The Exercise Option

In the early years of research investigating the exercise and mental health relationship, self-concept was identified as the psychological variable with the greatest potential to be improved. Because body image is intimately connected to our self-image, it is not surprising to find that when our body image improves through exercise, there is frequently an improvement in our self-image as well.

This makes sense, since if we feel better about our appearance and conditioning, these feelings will improve our overall self-concept. You will recall that earlier in this chapter, self-concept was shown to be formed by adding up several more specific self-concepts. In this case, our body image is improved, thereby improving our overall self-concept.

There appears to be a fair amount of research to support this position. In fact, in preparing my previous book, *Foundations of Exercise and Mental Health*, I found over 50 specific experiments conducted around the world that examined the effects of exercise on self-concept. Almost 60% of these studies reported significant improvements when the participants were involved in an ongoing exercise program. This percentage improvement would compare favorably with the more traditional treatments discussed earlier. There is also every reason to believe that the success rate could be even higher if we attempt to match the exercise to the particular aspect of self-concept that needs improving. Previous research has imposed a particular type of exercise on the participants, with no consideration of their particular needs. While this approach has proven successful, consider how much more effective it would be if we first identified the area of self-concept that needed improvement, then matched an appropriate exercise that would best result in improvements in that specific area.

For example, if a person has a negative body image because of excess weight, it would be important to prescribe an exercise program that is most effective for weight loss. Improving this person's cardiovascular conditioning would do little good in changing the negative body image. On the other hand, a person who has been noticing a shortness of breath with minimal physical activity would need a somewhat different type of exercise aimed at general conditioning.

You will be provided with all the information you need to know on this topic later in the chapter. The important thing for you to remember at this point is that exercise can, indeed, improve your overall self-concept.

How Exercise Improves Self-Concept

In contrast to depression (chapter 3) and anxiety (chapter 4), very little research has attempted to explain the exercise and self-concept relationship. In fact, not one study has attempted to relate improvements in self-concept to the endorphin, monoamine, or thermogenic hypotheses. This is probably because there is no evidence that self-concept has a biochemical origin, as was the case with depression and anxiety.

Similarly, the distraction theory appears of limited value in aiding our understanding of the relationship between exercise and self-concept. In the case of depression or anxiety, a distracting activity, such as exercise, helps take the participant's mind off disturbing thoughts, thereby making him or her feel better. This doesn't appear to be the case with self-concept.

The most likely explanation for this difference is that self-concept represents a psychological *trait* rather than a state and, as such, is far more resistant to change due to a distracting activity. For this reason, we need to examine somewhat different types of explanations for how exercise can improve our self-concept.

Way back in chapter 1, you read about a theory called self-efficacy and saw how it explained the relationship between exercise and mental health. This concept of self-efficacy is probably the best explanation for how exercise can improve your overall self-concept.

Perhaps the best way to define self-efficacy is as a "situation-specific form of self-confidence." To paraphrase, self-efficacy really refers to the level and strength of our belief that we can successfully perform a given task. Before we engage in a behavior, we ask ourselves two questions. First, "Can I do this particular activity?" and second, "If I can, will I be successful?" Our answer to these questions will greatly influence our choice of activities, the amount of effort we will expend, and the degree of persistence we will show in sticking with that activity.

It is especially interesting to note that research has consistently shown that exercise can improve a participant's self-efficacy. If exercise can improve self-efficacy, and self-efficacy is a situation-specific form of self-confidence, it is tempting to suggest that self-efficacy is the reason that exercise is effective in improving self-concept.

If this is the case, it provides us with a specific implication. For our self-efficacy to be improved, we need to be successful at the activity. For this reason, it is important to approach exercise in small steps. This will provide the best opportunity for successful early experiences with exercise.

And finally, perhaps the simplest way to explain how an exercise program can improve self-concept is by providing the participant with a sense of accomplishment from confronting a difficult physical and psychological task (the exercise program) and mastering it. This feeling of accomplishment is likely responsible for the improved self-concept that results. For this reason, let's now turn our attention to those features of an exercise program with the most potential to improve our overall level of self-concept.

What Exercises Are Best?

Picking a physical activity is the first step in the exercise for improved self-concept process. At this point you are undoubtedly wondering if there is an ideal exercise, or if some exercises are better than others for changing the way we feel about ourselves. Although a wide range of activities has been studied, two exercises in particular have consistently been associated with improved self-concept. The following guideline summarizes this research.

Exercise Guideline 2.1
Jogging is the physical activity that has most often been associated with improved self-concept in the participant. In fact, a large majority of studies have employed this type of exercise. The second most popular exercise for improving self-image appears to be weight lifting.

However, just because these two activities have been studied the most does not mean that they are the only ones with potential to improve our self-concept. For this reason, it is important to look at studies that have attempted to compare different types of exercise in terms of their beneficial effects.

In one experiment,[1] 40 women were randomly assigned to a running, weight-lifting, or nonexercise group. Results indicated that both exercise groups experienced improved self-concept, with the weight-lifting group showing slightly better results.

A similar study[2] compared the effects of swimming and weight lifting on self-concept in 89 male and female college students. The results of this study indicated that only the weight-lifting group enjoyed improved self-concept. The authors of this study proposed an interesting explanation for this finding. They suggested that overall self-concept may be tied to the participant's perceptions of his or her body and physical appearance and that weight lifting has the greatest potential to change physical appearance.

Although this is a good idea, it is also somewhat misleading. A better explanation may be that certain activities will be more appropriate for some individuals, but not for others. This is because the exercise program likely has to be chosen on the basis of the participant's goals. In other words, the exercise program should be tailored to the individual's needs.

Exercise Guideline 2.2
It is likely that the appropriate exercise for any one person will depend on the participant's initial physical appearance and perceived area of needed improvement. For example, running or walking may be more effective for people wishing to lose weight or improve their overall fitness level. Weight lifting, on the other hand, may be a wiser choice for anyone who is somewhat thin or someone who wishes to improve his or her musculature.

The key thing to remember is that you should ask yourself what exactly it is that you want to improve. Then pick an exercise with the best potential to meet that need. If you want to lose weight, pick a physical activity that you can perform slowly for a relatively long period of time. This will allow you to burn more calories. If you want bigger muscles, choose weight lifting. The resistance that comes from lifting weights will help develop your muscles. If you want to strengthen your heart and circulatory system, jogging, cycling, swimming, or aerobic dance would probably all serve your needs. These activities will provide sufficient intensity effort to improve your cardiovascular fitness.

Is Competition a Good Idea?

This is a difficult question to answer because different people have different needs. For some, especially those who have exercised regularly for several years, the element of competition can add spice to their exercise program. For others, however, especially those who are relatively new to regular exercise, this may not be the case. Competition for these individuals may have an undesirable effect.

Exercise Guideline 2.3
Recent research suggests it may be wise to avoid including a competitive element in the exercise program. Competitive conditions, especially when they result in a losing outcome, have actually had a negative effect on the participant's self-concept.

Intuitively, this guideline makes a good deal of sense. Winning makes us feel better about ourselves, while losing makes us feel worse. The problem with this situation is that if we are competing against another individual, one person always has to lose. For this reason, if you feel that you really want to include some competition in your exercise program, why not set realistic goals and then compete *against yourself?* For example, challenge yourself to go just a few more minutes on your next walk. This will greatly improve your chances of a "winning" outcome.

Some well-designed research lends support to this position. In one study,[3] 137 girls aged 11 through 14 years were divided into three groups. In the first group, the girls formed pairs, then cooperated to complete the physical exercises. In the second group, the girls competed to see who could perform the most exercises in a period of time. The third group was asked to exercise in a setting where there was neither cooperation nor competition.

At the conclusion of this study, only the cooperative group showed improvements in self-concept. More important, the competitive group actually experienced reduced self-concept. This finding does not speak well for the inclusion of competition in your exercise program.

A similar finding was reported in a study[4] that divided 24 male and female college students into three groups. The first group participated in a compete-win situation, while a second group was involved in a compete-lose scenario. A third group was assigned to noncompetitive tasks. At the conclusion of the experiment, the compete-lose group showed worsened self-concept.

When both of these studies are taken together, it appears that competition may actually defeat your purpose in an exercise program.

How Often Should I Exercise?

Now that you have chosen an exercise that you feel would be best suited for your purposes, it is important to determine how often it must be performed to get the best results. Fortunately, research provides a suitable answer to this question.

Exercise Guideline 2.4

Exercise frequencies of four or more times per week appear most effective in improving self-concept. It is important to note, however, that exercising more than three times per week is not recommended for most people, especially if their initial fitness levels are low. If you feel this is the case in your particular situation, it is advisable to stick to three exercise sessions per week and attempt to prolong your program. Another possibility is to choose a low-intensity exercise, such as walking; then you can feel safe exercising four or five times a week.

Regardless of the type of exercise you have chosen, it is a good idea to start slowly, then work up to more sessions once your body has had a chance to adapt to the physical activity. If you prefer a harder type of workout, such as jogging, swimming, or aerobic dance, then there is no reason that you will ever need to exercise more than three times per week. Remember, though, your choice of physical activity should be determined by your own needs, and not by the number of sessions that it will be necessary to perform each week.

How Hard Should I Exercise?

For some reason, only a few research studies have reported the exercise intensities that were used in their programs.

Exercise Guideline 2.5
Because of the lack of information provided in the research, it is not possible to state with certainty how hard you must exercise to experience the benefits of improved self-concept. For this reason, it is strongly recommended that you employ only mild to moderate exercise intensities. This is especially true if you are just beginning an exercise program or have been involved for only a short time.

When you get right down to it, this exercise guideline can be seen as good news. It suggests that there is no reason for you to be uncomfortable during your workouts. It means that a more leisurely, and hence more enjoyable, pace of activity will be every bit as effective as a strenuous session.

This makes sense when you recall our earlier discussion regarding choosing an appropriate exercise. Unless you want to improve your cardiovascular system as a main goal, higher-intensity exercise is not necessary. Even if this is an important goal for you, some recent research suggests that lower-intensity exercises performed for longer periods of time can be effective in improving your fitness level.

How Long Should I Exercise?

So far, every exercise guideline in this chapter has provided you with good news. In this case, however, there is no easy way out.

Exercise Guideline 2.6
When all of the research is examined, it appears that exercise sessions of approximately one hour are most often associated with improvements in self-concept. This is somewhat misleading, however, since in almost all cases, this one-hour period included warm-up and cool-down sessions. In fact, in most cases, the actual exercise sessions usually involved only 30 minutes. For this reason, it is advisable to try to work your way up to exercise sessions that are a minimum of 30 minutes in duration.

It is interesting to speculate as to why exercise sessions must be so long to be effective. Perhaps the best explanation relates to our earlier discussion on how changes in our self-concept are brought about by changes in body image. For example, if your goal is to lose weight, it is necessary to exercise at a mild or moderate intensity for a prolonged period of time. This will tax the correct systems in your body and allow you to burn more calories. Many experts believe that a 30- to 40-minute walk will burn more fat than will a 15-minute jog. Also, because walking is less strenuous, you can do it for longer periods of time. This will allow you to lose more weight and hence feel better about yourself.

A similar argument applies to working out with weights. When your goal is to improve your musculature, it is necessary to spend a good deal of time in the weight room. This is because you will have to perform several sets of several more repetitions (see chapter 5) to achieve the desired muscular development. If you have ever worked out with weights, you will already know that you have to spend a fair amount of time recuperating between sets. For this reason, the actual length of your exercise sessions will be longer than they would be for other types of exercise. Few people will complete a weight-lifting workout in less than 45 minutes to one hour.

How Soon Will I See Improvement?

Because self-concept represents a relatively stable and enduring trait, it stands to reason that an exercise program must be performed over a prolonged period to bring about the desired changes. Completed research supports this statement.

Exercise Guideline 2.7
Exercise programs involving 12 weeks or more of participation almost always result in significant improvements in self-concept. This indicates that the program must be of sufficient length to bring about changes in cardiovascular fitness, body composition, and muscular development.

Experimental support for this guideline is provided by a study involving 108 female college students. These individuals engaged in different types of exercise, including aerobic dance, jogging, swimming, and weight lifting. Exercise was performed three times per week for 60 minutes a session. At the end of the eight-week program, none of the exercise groups demonstrated improved self-concept. This finding was somewhat surprising, since all of these activities have been associated with improved self-concept in other studies. The authors concluded that the exercise program was not performed for a long enough period to produce changes in the participants' self-concepts. They further predicted that if the study had been prolonged for several more weeks, this would have provided enough time to bring about the desired changes. This viewpoint is supported by the fact that most research studies using exercise programs of greater than 12 weeks also report improvements in self-concept. It therefore appears that a minimum of 12 weeks is necessary for exercise to improve our body images and hence our self-concepts.

Some Final Helpful Hints

Remember to match your choice of exercise to your personal goals.

This might be the most important hint of all. Earlier in this chapter, it was pointed out that our exercise preference should take into consideration what it is that we would like to improve about ourselves. It is important to remember that certain exercises are good for some things, while other types of exercise are better for others.

Take a few minutes to review the section on "what exercises are best." Keep in mind that exercise will prove effective in improving your self-concept if you match the exercise to your needed area of development.

Be patient.

Don't expect immediate results. Your self-concept didn't develop overnight, so it isn't likely to improve overnight either. Remember, exercise takes time to bring about bodily changes. This is likely the main reason that exercise programs must be performed at least 12 weeks before improvements in self-concept occur. So take your time, learn to enjoy your activity, and everything else will fall into place.

Set reasonable and achievable goals.

It is always a good idea to set several smaller goals rather than one or more larger ones. In other words, if you want to lose 20 pounds, it is better to set weekly goals of one pound per week and have a weekly "weigh-in" rather than get on the scales once every 10 weeks and hope for larger weight losses of 10 or more pounds. The reason for this is simple. It allows you to build on success, and the rewards are more noticeable more often. In other words, you can earn 20 mental "pats on the back" if you lose only one pound at each of your weekly weigh-ins. On the other hand, setting a goal to lose 10 pounds by your next trip to the scales is a daunting prospect. So remember, take "baby steps" and build on success. This is the best recipe for improved self-concept through exercise.

If you must compete, compete only with yourself.

Earlier in this chapter, you read how competition, especially when you lose, can actually lead to a lower self-concept. So, unless you are one of those rare individuals who actually thrive on both the thrill of victory *and* the agony of defeat, it is best to avoid competing with a workout partner. If you want to stoke your competitive fires, why not compete against yourself by setting goals that are achievable and then challenging yourself to reach these goals?

Use positive self-statements regularly.

Much research suggests that how we think often determines how we feel. Most of us can easily identify with this viewpoint. Think back to the last time you woke up in the morning and said to yourself, "This is going to be a rotten day." Almost without exception, the prediction comes true. This is probably because you are setting up what the researchers call a self-fulfilling prophecy. In other words, you see what you think you are going to see. Fortunately, this same process can also work to your advantage if you use more appropriate statements. When working out, use positive self-statements, such as, "Way to go — you're looking good," or, "Great workout — this is feeling better all the time." Positive self-statements such as these can go a long way in helping exercise improve your self-concept.

Review chapters 5 and 6 before starting your program.

Before proceeding further, use the guidelines provided in chapter 5 to determine if exercise is safe for you. You will also find it helpful to review the different types of exercise. This will help you match the type of activity to your particular needs. You should also take the time to read chapter 6. This will provide all the help you need in sticking with your exercise program.

Looking Back

In chapter 2, you learned how self-concept is believed to be the best indicator of overall emotional adjustment. Low self-concept has been linked to depression, anxiety, substance abuse, and a variety of other problems. For this reason, the development of a positive self-concept is of utmost importance. Early in the chapter, you were encouraged to go through the Low Self-Concept Checklist as a self-awareness exercise. You were then shown how exercise has the potential to improve your overall self-concept. It now appears that exercise does this by improving your self-efficacy, or situation-specific self-confidence. The good feeling you get after completing an exercise session is a good example of this process. In terms of the actual exercises themselves, you were encouraged to ask yourself what you would most like to get out of an exercise program, then pick an activity that has the best potential to meet your needs. You should exercise a minimum of four times per week for approximately 30 minutes per session at a mild or moderate intensity. If you follow these guidelines, you can expect to see improvement in approximately 12 weeks.

Note

1. Ossip-Klein, D.J., Doyne, E.J., Bowman, E.D., Osborn, K.M., McDougal-Wilson, J.B., & Neimeyer, R.A. (1989). Effects of running or weight lifting on self-concept in clinically depressed women. *Journal of Consulting and Clinical Psychology, 57*, 158–161.

2. Stein, P.N., & Motta, R.W. (1992). Effects of aerobic and nonaerobic exercise on depression and self-concept. *Perceptual and Motor Skills, 74*, 79–89.

3. Marsh, H.W., & Peart, N.D. (1988). Competitive and co-operative physical fitness training programs for girls: Effects on physical fitness and multi-dimensional self-concepts. *Journal of Sport and Exercise Psychology, 10*, 390–407.

4. Caruso, C.M., Dzewaltowski, P.A., Gill, D.L., & McElroy, M.A. (1990). Psychological and physiological changes in competitive state anxiety during noncompetition and competitive success and failure. *Journal of Sport and Exercise Psychology, 2*, 6–20.

CHAPTER 3

FIGHTING DEPRESSION WITH EXERCISE

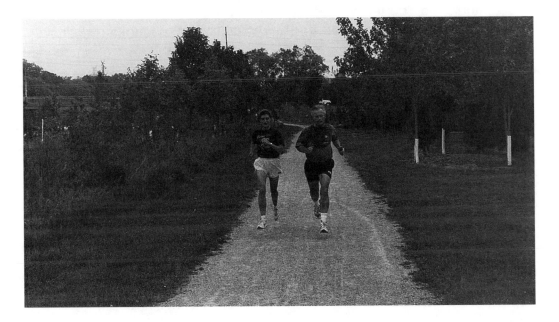

Now is the time to take back some control over your depressing thoughts. I'm sure you will be happy to hear that this new technique costs little or no money, can be done on your own time, and results in many additional benefits.

In this chapter, we will
- ✓ examine the mood called depression.
- ✓ learn how to recognize depression.
- ✓ discuss traditional treatments.
- ✓ provide you with a new and exciting way to fight back.
- ✓ discover what exercises are best to fight depression.
- ✓ learn how often, how hard, and how long you have to exercise to get the beneficial effects.
- ✓ provide a time frame for noticeable improvement.

How Common Is Depression?

Depression is a mood state experienced by almost everyone at some time. As we deal with the daily frustrations and stressors of modern living, it is natural to experience temporary mood swings. If we are lucky, this day-to-day type of depression lasts for only a short time, then goes away on its own. In other cases, called clinical depression, these feelings represent a much more lasting and serious problem, often requiring medical intervention.

A major study performed by the National Institute of Mental Health has reported that depression is the third most prevalent psychological disorder, afflicting approximately 6% of the American population (9.4 million people). When we add to this number the many more individuals who experience normal, or nonclinical depression, we begin to see how common the problem of depression is.

As a point of reference, let's now turn our attention to the symptoms of depression. This will help you identify the early warning signs, as well as the nature and extent of the problem.

How Can I Recognize Problems with Depression?

In terms of clinical depression, it is generally accepted that a Major Depressive Episode involves either a depressed mood or a loss of interest or pleasure in all or most activities, and the presence of other associated symptoms for at least a two-week period. These symptoms must be persistent and represent a marked change from previous functioning. In addition, at least five of the nine symptoms shown in the following checklist must be present.

Read through the checklist on the following page, and check off those symptoms that you are experiencing. This will help you determine your own degree of depression. Remember, depression doesn't have to be caused by life events. If you are depressed, but cannot identify situational factors that may be causing your depression, you may have endogenous depression. Problems of this nature are caused by internal, unknown causes, such as a chemical imbalance in the brain.

Regardless of the causes of your depression, remember, if you are experiencing a depressed mood or a loss of interest in all or most activities *and* notice at least five of the symptoms on the following checklist, you are advised to seek medical advice.

Of course, problems with depression are by no means restricted to the psychiatric population. As we discussed earlier, nonclinical depression is experienced by almost all of us at some time. In most cases, depression of this nature is usually tied to troubling events in our immediate environment. The most common causes usually involve grief or loss. In some cases, this loss is job-related. Common examples would include termination of employment, transfer to another location, failure to be promoted, or even retirement. A somewhat different type of loss involves some form of separation. The death of a pet, a jilted romance, or leaving home to live on your own are all examples of separation that may cause depression.

DEPRESSION CHECKLIST	
Loss of appetite	_____
Weight loss or gain	_____
Disturbance of sleep patterns	_____
Psychomotor retardation or agitation	_____
Decrease in energy	_____
Sense of worthlessness	_____
Guilt	_____
Difficulty in concentrating	_____
Thoughts of suicide	_____

Finally, some individuals become depressed when they complete an important project, such as graduating from university, getting their first job, or moving into their "dream home." While you would normally expect people to be happy in situations such as these, the reaching of an important goal is usually anticlimactic and involves a letdown. People often question the amount of time and effort expended once the goal has been reached. This is probably because the eager anticipation that has been the driving force is no longer there to motivate them.

In most of these instances, brief periods of depression are normal and subside on their own after a few days. It is only when these depressive episodes become frequent, severe, and long-lasting that we suffer from a mood disorder that could be considered clinical.

How Is Depression Usually Treated?

As mentioned earlier, nonclinical depression almost always subsides after a brief period without medical intervention. People should seek medical advice, however, if they feel they are suffering from clinical depression.

One of the earliest treatments for depression is psychotherapy. Most experts agree that this type of "talking-out therapy" is moderately helpful. It also appears that different types of psychotherapy are equally effective. As a general guideline, even though psychotherapy is often effective with mild and moderate depression, it is frequently supplemented with antidepressive medications. Cases of severe depression almost always require medication.

Traditionally, the most widely prescribed medications are tricyclic antidepressants. Most common among this family of drugs would be Surmontil, Elavil, and Tofranil. Although these medications produce results within about three weeks, they also have their down side. Tricyclic medication often produces side effects, such as blurred vision, dry mouth, and orthostatic hypotension (dizziness when standing up suddenly).

If patients fail to respond to tricyclic antidepressants, they are sometimes prescribed monoamine oxidase inhibitors, especially Nardil, Parnate, and Marplan. As with the previous class of drugs, this type is also accompanied by serious side effects, such as dangerous interactions with certain foods and other drugs, hypertension, and irregular heart rate and rhythm. For this reason, the monoamine oxidase inhibitors are usually prescribed as a last-resort medication.

Recently, many medical practitioners are prescribing Prozac as a first-line treatment of depression. So far, the results look promising, especially in view of the infrequent and mild side effects. Of course, since the drug is relatively new, it will be several years before we know the exact nature and severity of side effects.

One final category of depression deserves mention. So far, all of the preceding treatments have focused on unipolar (mood downswing only) depression. Another illness called bipolar affective disorder (also known as manic-depression) also shows symptoms of mood downswing as well as mood upswing (mania). Traditional treatment for this illness almost always involves lithium medication, since nothing else has worked better. As with other drugs, lithium also has some problematic side effects. Most noticeable among these are lethargy, poor muscular coordination, and fine hand tremor. In addition, long-term use has sometimes been associated with kidney and thyroid problems. Recently, some doctors have been prescribing anticonvulsive medications, such as Tegretol and Valproic Acid, to control bipolar affective disorder. The effectiveness of this latter category of drug will be determined over time. In all cases, individuals using these drugs should seek medical guidance.

In summary, the relatively long time frame required for psychotherapy, as well as the disturbing side effects of the various medications, highlights the need for a supplemental form of treatment. The remainder of this chapter will focus on the potential of exercise to serve this valuable function.

The Exercise Option

During the past 20 years, a substantial body of research has accumulated demonstrating the potential of exercise to lower depression in the participant.

A major study conducted in the United States[1] has investigated the relationship between physical activity patterns and well-being in several thousand U.S. and Canadian households. The results of this study indicate that regular exercise is associated with positive mood, general well-being, and relatively infrequent symptoms of depression and stress.

One of my previous books certainly supports this position. After reviewing almost 50 different experiments from around the world, the most important fact that emerged was that over 80% of these studies report significant reductions in depression following exercise. Although these studies were completed independently and involved a wide range of participants, when taken together they highlight the potential of exercise to lower participant depression. The following case portrays a likely scenario.

Dave's Divorce

Dave just couldn't believe it. After 15 years of marriage, his wife had just told him she was filing for divorce. Although their marriage had been far from perfect, it came as a tremendous shock to be served with the papers. His wife had moved out three months previously, telling him she needed some time to sort things out. Two months after the decree was signed, Dave quit his job and left town. Dave had always enjoyed working in the department store, but looked forward to his newfound freedom. Unfortunately, though, this freedom provided little satisfaction, and he became increasingly more depressed in the six weeks before his self-referral. For the last few of these weeks, Dave had trouble getting to sleep every night, had little appetite, felt very tired, and showed no interest in his usual activities. He had seen his family doctor and had been given a small number of sleeping pills. The night before calling for his appointment, he found himself thinking just how easy it would be to take all the pills along with a few stiff drinks. Fortunately, at this point, Dave decided that life had far too much to offer to check out now. The next morning, he phoned his family doctor and made an appointment with a psychiatrist. After the first few sessions, he was told that antidepressant medications, such as Prozac, would probably be of little value in his case, and he should try a more proactive approach such as exercise. As it turned out, this was the best advice he had received in years. Although Dave used to jog regularly, he hadn't done so in over a year. After 10 weeks of getting back into jogging 20 minutes, three times per week, Dave noticed a marked improvement in his mood and promised himself he would stick with his exercise program.

Exercise has also been shown to be effective for individuals who are clinically depressed. A recent study conducted in Norway[2] best supports these results. Forty-three patients who had been treated in a hospital for major depression were interviewed one to two years after their discharge. Each person was asked to evaluate the different types of therapy received while at the mental health clinic. The different therapies included antidepressant medication, community meetings, contact with other patients, group psychotherapy, individual psychotherapy, physical exercise, and contact with staff. Patients ranked physical exercise as the most important element in their overall treatment program. This finding suggests that exercise may be an important treatment component for depressed patients.

Can Exercise Prevent Depression?

In the early years of research on this important topic, the experts seemed to feel that exercise was effective only as a treatment for depression. For this reason, most of the studies involved individuals who were being treated for depression as either inpatients or outpatients at mental health clinics. As you have already seen in the preceding section, these people found exercise to be highly effective in treating symptoms of depression.

At this point, the research focus shifted to include those individuals who were not clinically depressed, but still showed some of the symptoms of depression. Examples included a group of patients who had recently suffered a heart attack, males with chronic obstructive pulmonary disease, alcoholics, hypertensive male adults, premenopausal females, and adults who were depressed but not clinically so. In all of these cases, the individuals scored higher on tests of depression, but not high enough to require medical help. Even so, participation in a regular exercise program repeatedly lowered the overall level of depression in these participants as well. At this point, researchers concluded that as long as the participant shows symptoms of depression, exercise can be an effective treatment.

Since research usually builds upon past findings, the next logical step was to determine the effect of exercise on individuals who were not reporting any symptoms of depression. To do this, research was performed with male and female college students, male and female healthy adults, and older adults. In all of these cases, the participants scored in the "normal" range of depression prior to their exercise program. In other words, they did not experience any obvious symptoms of depression. At the conclusion of their prescribed exercise programs, an interesting finding emerged. These participants also showed significantly lower depression scores than they had during the initial testing, even though they were not depressed to begin with.

At this point, you are probably wondering how you can reduce depression in someone who is not experiencing any of the symptoms of depression. Perhaps the best way to explain this occurrence is to use the analogy of blood pressure. When you go to your family doctor and have your blood pressure taken, he or she will tell you whether or not you are in the normal range. If your reading is outside the normal range, you will be told that some changes are needed. If your blood pressure is in the normal range, however, no adjustments are required. This does not mean, however, that your blood pressure can't be changed. By eliminating excess salt from your diet and participating in regular exercise, you can lower your blood pressure to an even better reading. This same situation holds for depression scores. Even though a person scores in the normal range for depression, his or her depression score can still be reduced.

This outcome is important. It suggests that participants can actually lower their "baseline" depression by participating in a regular exercise program. By starting from a lower baseline, regular exercise may, in fact, serve the function of preventing depression from occurring in the first place. Although research has not yet established this connection, there is every reason to believe it will do so in the near future. Obviously, preventing depression is always preferable to treating it. Exercise may have the potential to do just that.

Regardless of whether you want to use exercise to treat depression or attempt to prevent it from happening, there are certain things you need to know about the exercise itself. The following sections will provide all the important information you need to get started using exercise in the battle against depression.

How Exercise Fights Depression

The fact that exercise consistently reduces depression in the participant has led researchers to speculate as to the cause of this relationship. At present, several explanations appear reasonable.

Chapter 1 introduced possible ways that exercise could influence mental health. In this section, we will look only at those arguments specific to depression.

One possible way that exercise fights depression involves the release of endorphins. You will recall that endorphins are the body's "feel-good" chemicals. A substantial body of research has shown that exercise causes an elevation in blood plasma endorphin levels. In one study,[3] seven untrained females volunteered to participate in an increasingly intense exercise program for two months. After exercising for an hour a day, six days per week, these women had endorphin levels that rose from 57% above normal during the first week to 145% above normal by the end of two months. Other studies have reported similar results. Since endorphins are the body's normal mood-enhancing drug, it is possible that exercise reduces depression by causing more of these "feel-good" chemicals to be present in our bloodstreams. Although this provides a possible explanation, it still has not been conclusively proven.

A more widely accepted explanation suggests that improvements in depression are the result of exercise's altering one or more of the major brain monoamines (i.e., dopamine, serotonin, and norepinephrine). Evidence for this theory comes from studies that demonstrate that these chemicals are markedly reduced in depressed patients. In fact, experts now agree that depression is caused by an impaired transmission of these chemicals along certain neural pathways of the brain. Of special interest to us is the finding that exercise appears to increase the levels and transmission capabilities of these chemicals.

By restoring the proper balance of monoamines, it is thought that exercise has the effect of reducing depression.

So far, we have considered only biochemical explanations for the effect of exercise on depression. A somewhat different line of thinking suggests that psychological factors may also be at work. Many people believe that exercise has been effective against depression because of its potential to distract the participant. Endurance athletes, in particular, have reported that it is virtually impossible to train long and hard and be depressed. Because the athletes are concentrating on thoughts such as their training goals and the physical sensations of the workouts, it is likely that their minds are taken off depressing and troubling thoughts. As long as these athletes do not train excessively to the point of staleness and burnout, they appear to enjoy a type of resistance to depression. This same argument holds for the recreational exerciser, whose main goal is to finish the workout before running out of breath. In both of these cases, exercise may be effective because it serves as a type of distraction from depressing thoughts. In other words, it provides us with an effective time-out, giving us something else to think about.

A final explanation relates to self-efficacy and skills mastery. Most therapists maintain that to reduce depression, regardless of the type of therapy, the following conditions must be met: (a) The patients must be provided with a plan of action, helping them believe they can control their own behavior; (b) the patients must be taught specific skills to cope with depression; (c) the ability to use these new skills independently to attain the desired goal is necessary; and (d) the patients must come to believe that the improved mood is the result of learning this new skill. Looking at this list, I'm sure you will agree that participation in a regular exercise program, as outlined in this chapter, incorporates all of the necessary ingredients. Perhaps exercise reduces depression simply by providing a feeling of self-confidence. This feeling likely stems from the awareness that a particular exercise has been mastered, and you have followed through with your program.

In summary, a variety of theories have been presented to explain how exercise can help fight depression. The most likely scenario is that several of these explanations work together to produce the desired results. Until research sheds more light on the exact nature of this relationship, we can take comfort in just knowing that exercise is an effective behavior for both preventing and treating depression.

What Exercises Are Best?

By now, you probably have several questions regarding the use of exercise to prevent or treat depression. The first question that invariably comes to mind is, "What exercise will produce the best results?" Although research has not yet identified one particular exercise as superior in terms of its potential to reduce depression, it has identified several different types of exercise that will do the job.

> ### Exercise Guideline 3.1
> **Walking and jogging are the two exercises that have been most consistently associated with reduced depression in the participant. In addition to these two activities, cycling, aerobic dance, and weight lifting have also been shown to be effective.**

Research experiments have compared the effect of different exercises on depression. In one study,[4] a group of joggers was compared to a group of weight lifters. All participants were healthy, nondepressed females. The results indicated that both groups experienced significantly lower depression after exercise. In addition, neither activity was superior to the other in terms of beneficial effects.

Although research has failed to identify the one "perfect exercise" for depression, it has provided us with some important answers and implications. All of the exercises we have discussed appear to have two common elements. They involve the large muscle groups (arms, legs, and torso) and are rhythmic in nature. Any exercise that meets these two criteria will probably be effective in reducing depression.

This finding provides a very important implication. Since a variety of exercises appear to be equally effective, this means that you have the opportunity to pick the exercise that you like best. This is always much better than being told what you have to do. You will also find it much easier to stick with an exercise program if you have picked the exercise yourself. So go back to the first exercise guideline and see which activity has the most appeal for you personally. More information on these exercises is provided in chapter 5.

How Often Should I Exercise?

Once you have chosen the particular type of exercise that you would like to perform, the next logical question is, "How often do I have to exercise to get results?" Completed research provides us with a suitable answer to that question.

Exercise Guideline 3.2
Exercise performed three times per week appears sufficient to significantly reduce depression. Although improvements have also been noted with greater exercise frequencies, there does not appear to be any added advantage to exercising more than three or four times per week. By staying within this recommended range, you will reduce the risk of overuse injuries. You will also find it easier to stick with your program.

When we look at all the research that has been conducted on this topic, it appears that exercise will reduce depression provided you exercise at least three times per week. When exercise is performed less often, the cumulative effects of the exercise may not be sufficient to reduce depression. On the other hand, exercising too often (i.e., daily) may also fail to produce beneficial results. This is likely because we view the number of exercise sessions per week as excessive. When this happens, exercise loses its mood-enhancing effect and may even actually become a stressful activity. If this happens, depression might actually increase rather than decrease.

The only notable exception to this guideline relates to the type of exercise. For example, if you choose walking as your preferred activity, it would be possible to perform this activity on an almost daily basis, provided you go about it at an easy pace and don't tire yourself out. Even so, most experts would recommend at least one day off, even if you do choose walking as the activity of choice. Obviously, the more strenuous activities, such as jogging, aerobic dance, and weight lifting, should be performed less frequently.

How Hard Should I Exercise?

When many people think of exercise, they conjure up images of exhaustion, heavy breathing, sore muscles, sweating, and tedium. Fortunately, if we are using exercise to improve our mental health, we don't really need to exercise that hard.

Exercise Guideline 3.3
Research indicates that both high- and moderate-intensity exercise have similar effects in lowering participant depression. Some studies also suggest that even mild-intensity exercise can produce the same results. For this reason, it seems logical to exercise at a moderate- or even mild-intensity level since the effects appear the same, yet pose less risk of injury and discomfort.

This is certainly good news for most of us. An obvious implication, especially for those who are new to exercise, is to start easy. A good rule of thumb is that you should be able to carry on a normal conversation with your exercise partner, without running out of breath. If you can do this, you are probably exercising at a mild- to moderate-intensity level. This guideline is called the "talk-test," and is used by most individuals to guard against exercising too strenuously.

Remember, your exercise does not have to make you huff and puff to produce improvements in depression. The key is to get out and get active. If you do this, the results will look after themselves.

How Long Should I Exercise?

It isn't necessary to exercise for long periods of time to enjoy the benefits. In fact, when you look at the following guideline, you will see that the old excuse "I just don't have enough time to exercise" doesn't make sense.

Exercise Guideline 3.4
Exercise sessions lasting 15–30 minutes appear long enough to produce both physiological improvements and reduced depression.

This means that if you follow the earlier guideline and exercise three times per week, with each session lasting 15–30 minutes, your total amount of weekly exercise would be 45–90 minutes. Almost everyone can fit that amount of time into a busy schedule. If necessary, ask for help. For example, a mother working outside the home could ask her husband to look after the children for 25 to 30 minutes after supper so she could take a walk. Similarly, the business executive at work could fit in some exercise during lunch break.

Remember, if you want to exercise longer each session, go ahead. The guidelines we present in this chapter represent minimum requirements that will produce the desired psychological benefits.

How Soon Will I See Improvement?

Some individuals have reported improvement after their first workout. For most people, however, it takes a while before the effects of exercise become noticeable. This is probably because changes with exercise are cumulative, requiring a certain amount of time to appear.

Exercise Guideline 3.5
The majority of research studies demonstrating reductions in depression have involved exercise programs of at least 10 weeks in duration. Although some evidence exists that suggests improvements can occur with shorter exercise programs, the most consistent results are associated with the longer programs.

Although we should not expect lasting results for at least 10 weeks, even a single bout of exercise has the potential to reduce depression in the participant. This possibility is important. It suggests that exercise can be also be used as a Band-Aid approach to deal with daily depression and mood states. In other words, if a person is feeling down on a given day, one of the best responses is to get out and exercise. Going for a walk, a jog, or a bike ride, or lifting weights may be enough to chase away the blues.

Although exercise may be effective in reducing depression after one session, you would be well-advised to adopt exercise as one of your regular activities. It seems reasonable to believe that the longer the exercise program, the greater the chance that the changes in depression will be lasting. It also seems likely that participation in a regular exercise program has the best potential to prevent depression from occurring in the first place.

In summary, you will probably experience the best results if you follow a regular exercise program for at least 10 weeks. As an added bonus, however, feel free to use single exercise sessions to combat daily mood swings.

Some Final Helpful Hints

Learn to exercise when you need it most.

One of the most difficult tasks you may face is convincing yourself you should exercise when you are feeling depressed. This is one of the least likely times you want to get out and get active. For this reason, especially in the early stages of your exercise program, it is a good idea to adopt a "buddy system." By arranging to exercise with a friend, you are increasing your chances of participating, even on those days when you don't feel like it. Research indicates that you are less inclined to skip exercise sessions if someone else is depending on your company. This is probably because you would feel guilty about letting the other person down. Over time, once exercise has become part of your lifestyle, this social component may no longer be necessary. In the meantime, the companionship will give you the needed motivation and may even help improve your mood by providing enjoyable company. Other tools that will help you stick with your program in the initial stages are provided in chapter 6. Armed with this information, your chances of sticking with your program will be greatly improved.

Don't be swayed by a friend.

Another helpful hint is to make sure that *you* pick the type of exercise you want to perform. A variety of appropriate exercises was provided earlier in the chapter. Quite often, a person will join a friend who is already engaged in an ongoing program. While this can work well and is certainly easy, you have to be sure that the physical activity is one that you would choose for yourself. Otherwise, if you adopt a friend's preferred exercise and find you don't like it, you may find that your mood will actually worsen. No one benefits from performing a hated activity. For this reason, you are well-advised to select your own preferred type of exercise, then see if you can find someone who prefers the same type of activity.

Go slowly.

It is also important that you start slowly, especially if you are not an experienced exerciser. If you try to do too much too fast, you will become overly tired, sore, and probably disappointed. You may even drop out under the protests of your aching body. If this happens, you will likely notice that you feel even more depressed than before, since in your own mind you have failed at your exercise attempts. For this reason, make sure you refer to chapter 5 for sample exercise programs appropriate to your personal exercise history. Remember, if you take it slowly, your exercise experience will be far more positive and enjoyable.

Concentrate on the positive aspects of your exercise session.

What you think about while you exercise may also be important. If you keep in mind the fact that you are exercising to prevent or reduce depression, it would make little sense for you to dwell on depressing thoughts during your workout. If you find this happening, try to shift your attention to more pleasant thoughts, such as how the exercise is improving your fitness level. Self-statements, such as "I'm getting a good workout" or "Think happy thoughts," have also proven effective. The important thing is to find a word or phrase that works best for you. This will require some experimentation, but will be well worth your efforts.

It is also a good idea to have a plan that includes a variety of positive topics to think about once you have shifted your attention from negative thoughts. Some people like to mentally review favorite movies or former friendships. Others prefer to plan vacations or think about a memorable round of golf. Thought content of this nature is referred to as dissociative imagery by the experts and is very effective in improving your overall mood. Try implementing positive thought content in your workouts to supplement the positive benefits of exercise.

Read chapters 5 and 6 for more information.

Having read this chapter, you are in a much better position to use exercise in the fight against depression. Before you start to put these principles into action, make sure you read chapters 5 and 6. These chapters will (a) help you determine if exercise is safe for you, (b) provide you with a description of appropriate exercises, (c) outline sample programs for each exercise, and (d) show you how to stick with your program.

Looking Back

In this chapter, you learned that depression is a common and problematic mood state. You were then told how to recognize problems with depression and given the opportunity to complete a Depression Checklist. A variety of traditional treatments were then discussed, and you were able to consider the advantages and disadvantages of each approach. At this point, you were provided with another optional treatment — exercise. A variety of explanations for the depression-reducing effects of exercise were discussed. Some of these were biochemical, while others involved psychological interpretations. The most likely scenario is that a variety of these factors work together to produce the beneficial results. In terms of deciding which exercises work best, you saw how walking, jogging, cycling, aerobic dance, and weight lifting all proved to be effective. For this reason, you were encouraged to pick the activity you like best. Once you have done this, try to exercise a minimum of three times per week for 15 to 30 minutes per session at a moderate- or even mild-intensity level. Although you will probably notice an improvement in your mood after the first exercise session, the best and most lasting results will occur after you have followed your program for at least 10 weeks.

Note

1. Stephens, T. (1988). Physical and mental health in the United States and Canada: Evidence from four population surveys. *Preventive Medicine, 17*, 35–47.

2. Martinsen, E.W., & Medhus, A. (1989). Adherence to exercise and patients' evaluation of physical exercise in a comprehensive treatment programme for depression. *Nordisk-Psykiatrisk-Tidsskrift, 43*, 411–415.

3. Carr, D.B., Bullen, B.A., Skinrar, G., Arnold, M.A., Rosenblatt, M., Beitins, I.Z., Martin, J.B., & McArthur, J.W. (1981). Physical conditioning facilitates the exercised-induced secretion of Beta-endorphin and Beta-lipotropin in women. *The New England Journal of Medicine, 305*, 560–563.

4. Doyne, E.J., Ossip-Klein, D.J., Bowman, E.D., Osborn, K.M., McDougall-Wilson, J.B., & Neimeyer, R.A. (1987). Running versus weight lifting in the treatment of depression. *Journal of Consulting and Clinical Psychology, 55*, 748–754.

CHAPTER 4

COMBATING STRESS AND ANXIETY WITH EXERCISE

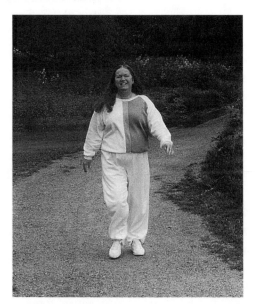

Almost every day of our lives, we face frustrating and stressful events. Although there is no way to avoid these unpleasant occurrences, how we deal with them is important in determining our overall level of physical and mental health. If we do not learn how to handle stress effectively, it will usually result in increased anxiety, along with physical ailments, such as high blood pressure, indigestion, and even ulcers. For this reason, it is important to have a game plan for coping with life's daily stressors.

After reading this chapter, you will have a whole new way of coping with daily stressors. This new technique is basically free, can be incorporated into your busy schedule, and has no undesirable side effects.

In this chapter, we will

✓ examine the mood called anxiety.

✓ learn how to recognize the symptoms.

✓ discuss traditional ways of dealing with anxiety.

✓ illustrate how exercise can make you feel better.

✓ look at what exercises are best to fight anxiety.

✓ learn how hard, how often, and how long we must exercise to obtain the mental health benefits.

✓ suggest a time frame for noticing improvements.

Is Stress the Same Thing as Anxiety?

Many people mistakenly use the terms *stress* and *anxiety* interchangeably. In reality, they refer to two very different concepts. Most experts agree that *stress* refers to a nonspecific response of the body to any demand made upon it. In other words, stress is a neutral (neither good nor bad) physiological response to some sort of stressor.

What this really means is that stress can be good just as much as it can be bad. Seeing your lottery numbers come up would be an example of good stress. A reprimand from your boss would be bad stress. The meaning we attribute to each of these stressors is what makes it either good or bad. It is our interpretation of the stressor, not the stressor itself, that results in positive or negative feelings.

For the most part, all of us are willing to take our chances with stressors of the lottery-win variety. It is the other types that we need to learn how to handle. When we interpret a stressor in a negative way (the boss's tongue-lashing), this causes worry, fear, and apprehension — the underpinnings of anxiety. *Anxiety*, then, is the negative emotion or mood state that we want to avoid as much as possible. In this chapter, you will learn how exercise has the potential to make you more resistant to the negative effects of daily stressors.

How Common Is Anxiety?

Occasional anxiety is a normal reaction to stress, and as long as it doesn't happen too often or too strongly, it is probably nothing to worry about. In most cases, it is simply an expected reaction to life's daily hassles, frustrations, expectations, and interpersonal relationships. For some people, however, the constant worry about real or imaginary problems can become so strong and so frequent that their anxiety reaches clinical proportions. When this happens, it often interferes with their work, family relationships, and overall health. It is advisable for these individuals to seek professional help.

Problems of this nature are by no means uncommon. Anxiety has been determined to be the most prevalent psychological disorder, affecting approximately 8% of the U.S. population. This represents a total of over 13.1 million people. And remember, this number does not include everyone else who experiences a normal range of day-to-day anxiety.

At this point, let's focus our attention on the symptoms of anxiety. This will help you determine if anxiety is a problem for you.

How Can I Recognize Problems with Anxiety?

Perhaps the best definition of anxiety is that it is a subjective feeling of apprehension and heightened physiological arousal. What this actually means is that the individual finds himself or herself worrying, as well as noticing a general feeling of physical unease.

In terms of clinical anxiety, a distinction must be made between phobic disorders and anxiety states. In phobic disorders, the person's concern or anxiety is directed toward a specific person or situation, such as spiders, snakes, dogs, or even open spaces. In contrast, anxiety states involve more generalized and less specific aspects of anxiety, such as unreasonable worry about getting through the day.

In some people, anxiety can occur suddenly, with little warning, and for no apparent reason. This most severe anxiety state is called *panic disorder*. This involves anxiety at its extreme — a very debilitating condition. It is recognizable by episodes of extreme anxiety and physical tension. Another central feature of panic disorder is what the experts call free-floating anxiety. This refers to anxiety with no apparent cause. The individual feels extremely anxious, but cannot tell what is causing the nervous feeling. And finally, some people experience a lower level of anxiety across a wider range of situations. This condition is called a *general anxiety disorder*, and is a long-term, less changeable version of panic disorder. In almost all cases, clinical anxiety should be treated by medical professionals.

As we have already mentioned, problems with anxiety are not restricted to the psychiatric population. Generalized, or subclinical anxiety, is experienced by almost everyone at some point in his or her life. The type of nervousness we experience before a job interview, an important exam, or a visit to the in-laws is referred to as *state anxiety*. In cases such as these, the symptoms appear shortly before the event and disappear almost immediately afterward. On the other hand, when the person experiences anxiety states very often and in a large variety of situations, this condition is called *trait anxiety*. Individuals who suffer from high trait anxiety are people who feel nervous much of the time, regardless of where they are or what they are doing. For these people, experiencing symptoms of anxiety has become a way of life.

Regardless of the type of anxiety you are experiencing, or the severity of the problem, the symptoms of anxiety remain relatively consistent. Read through the checklist on page 44 and mark those symptoms that you are experiencing on a regular basis. This will help you determine if anxiety is a problem for you and if you would benefit from this chapter.

Remember, all of us experience some of these symptoms occasionally. But if you find you are experiencing several on a regular basis, you are advised to read this chapter. This will allow you to discover a relatively simple remedy for dealing with daily stressors and anxiety.

ANXIETY CHECKLIST

Nervousness ____

Feeling of fear ____

Worry about the future ____

Sweating ____

Rapid heartbeat ____

Muscle tension ____

Headaches ____

Stomach cramps ____

Diarrhea ____

Shaky hands ____

How Is Anxiety Usually Treated?

For many people, these symptoms of anxiety usually disappear on their own within a short time. For other individuals, however, the problems do not go away on their own. When this happens, it is necessary to seek medical help to deal with the anxiety.

Traditionally, treatment for the anxiety states has included psychotherapy, cognitive therapy, and drug therapy. *Psychotherapy*, or "talking-out" therapy, has proven reasonably effective when the anxiety is a learned problem. In cases such as these, the individual has learned, or developed over time, anxiety-producing thoughts that are associated with certain people or events. Psychotherapy helps by teaching the person to block or replace the irrational thoughts that are causing the problem. By discussing the problem, the patient becomes aware of his or her faulty way of looking at real or anticipated events.

Recently, a somewhat different technique has helped many individuals. This process, known as *cognitive therapy*, attempts to change these faulty thought patterns that are causing the worry and anxiety.

This is done by helping the person recognize problem self-statements, such as "I'm a total failure," or "I just know that I am going to goof up," and then replace them with more realistic thoughts. In the previous two examples, more appropriate self-statements would be, "I'm not a total failure — everybody makes mistakes sometimes," and, "there is no reason to think I am going to goof up — I'm sure everything will turn out fine." By replacing the original faulty statements with more positive and realistic thoughts, the person is able to reduce or eliminate the problem anxiety.

Although psychotherapy has enjoyed a certain degree of success, and cognitive therapy has proven effective, their ultimate use by medical practitioners has been limited by two factors. First, it is difficult to know whether a person's anxiety is caused by faulty thinking or a somewhat different reason that involves biological causes. If the anxiety is learned, then there is every reason to believe that either psychotherapy or cognitive therapy could prove to be quite effective. If the anxiety is caused by biological or biochemical reasons, then psychotherapy will be of little use. Cognitive therapy, however, remains a valuable and effective treatment option. A second reason that these therapies have received limited use involves the difficulty in maintaining these strategies in everyday life, away from the therapist. Once the individual has left the treatment setting, it is easy to slip back into faulty ways of thinking. For this reason, drugs have been used most often as the front-line treatment for anxiety.

Drug therapy for anxiety usually involves minor tranquilizers. A drug family known as the benzodiazepines (e.g., Librium, Valium, Ativan, Dalmane, Xanax) represents the most often prescribed medications. The major advantages of these drugs are that they are highly effective and fast-acting. For example, drugs such as Ativan and Valium have proven to be effective in 70% to 80% of the users. In addition, the effects are usually felt within the first hour. It is easy to see, then, why these drugs would be a popular choice for both the patient and the doctor.

If the use of medication to control tension and anxiety seems too good to be true, then this is probably because it is. Using these drugs has serious disadvantages. First, this drug family has been widely abused, both by legal prescriptions as well as on the streets. Xanax, for example, is the third most widely prescribed drug in the United States. A second problem is that the prolonged use of these drugs usually results in physical dependence, more commonly called addiction. This results in symptoms of withdrawal when the medication is discontinued. This withdrawal usually involves flu-like symptoms, such as nausea, dizziness, fatigue, and extreme restlessness. These symptoms of withdrawal are often so severe that they seem as bad as or worse than the original anxiety. Finally, all of these drugs have been associated with serious side effects. These side effects usually involve problems such as skin reactions, dizziness, fainting, blurred vision, headache, nausea, disorientation, depression, disturbed sleep, dry mouth, and periodic amnesia.

While these side effects don't sound like much fun, the minor tranquilizers remain popular among users, probably because of their sedative, muscle-relaxing, and anxiety-reducing qualities. Clearly, however, a more positive and less problematic treatment supplement is needed. The rest of this chapter will show you how exercise has the potential to provide this alternative.

The Exercise Option

In 1988, a large study[1] was conducted in the United States and Canada. The purpose was to examine the relationship between the population's physical activity habits and their overall mental health. Almost 24,000 individuals took part in the project. The involvement of so many people strengthens our confidence in the overall findings.

Of major interest to this chapter is the finding that regular exercisers reported less frequent symptoms of anxiety and stress than was the case with less physically active people. As a bonus, this same group experienced a more positive overall mood and feeling of well-being.

In fact, quite a substantial amount of research supports this position. To gather information for my book, *Foundations of Exercise and Mental Health*, I reviewed almost 60 experiments conducted around the world that examined the relationship between exercise and anxiety. Almost 75% of these experiments reported significant reductions in anxiety when the participants had been involved in an exercise program. These findings, taken together, suggest that exercise has the potential to be used as an alternative or at least supplemental treatment for anxiety.

Researchers have attempted to test this theory, comparing exercise to other more traditional treatments for anxiety. The results of these studies are interesting, with the findings surprisingly consistent. For example, one particular study[2] employed aerobic dance as the exercise condition and another traditional treatment called autogenic relaxation training — a process that involves learning to relax your muscles. A third group engaged in quiet rest. As was the case with the first study, both the exercise group and the traditional relaxation-training group experienced greatly reduced anxiety. In this study, however, the quiet-rest group did not show improvement. Both anecdotal and experimental evidence seems to support our earlier viewpoint that exercise compares favorably to more traditional treatments for anxiety.

Some additional research has indicated that the reductions in anxiety resulting from exercise seem to last longer than is the case when more traditional treatments are used. As an added advantage, exercise is a less expensive process than are the other types of treatment. It also provides other health benefits. It therefore appears that you may wish to consider exercise as a valuable treatment alternative.

Can Exercise Make Us More Resistant to Stress?

There is also substantial evidence suggesting that exercise can actually make us more resistant to stress. In other words, it appears that individuals who exercise regularly are better able to deal with life's daily hassles. Although everyone is exposed to stressful situations, exercisers do not seem to experience the same degree of resulting anxiety as do nonexercisers. This is an important finding. By participating in a regular exercise program, we are actually preventing many of the problems associated with stress and anxiety. Preventing a problem is always a better alternative than treating it.

How Exercise Fights Anxiety

Although a wide range of explanations have been offered to explain how exercise can help fight anxiety, two of these appear to be accepted and logical. For this reason, we will now take a brief look at the thermogenic and distraction arguments introduced in chapter 1.

The thermogenic explanation, you will recall, relates to the idea of the body's warming with exercise. Early researchers consistently found that exercise resulted in decreased anxiety by reducing physical tension in the participants. These reductions in physical tension have been measured by means of changes in brain waves, reflexes, and muscular tension. Interestingly enough, these same physical changes can be produced by passively heating the body. This can be done by either turning up the temperature or using common techniques such as warm showers or sauna baths. Because exercise heats the body, and body warming produces a measurable relaxation effect, many experts believe this is how exercise reduces anxiety in the participant.

A second, somewhat different explanation involves a more psychological interpretation. The distraction hypothesis suggests that exercise reduces anxiety by providing the exerciser with a form of time-out from worrisome thoughts and events. This idea originated from the observation that resting quietly in an area free from distractions for 20 to 45 minutes actually resulted in lowered blood pressure and reduced anxiety. Exercise usually takes our minds off anxiety-provoking thoughts and other daily stressors. This in itself is enough to make us feel less anxious. Although this doesn't sound like a very scientific explanation, it still makes sense. When we continue to dwell on stressful thoughts, we are only making the situation worse. In fact, this whole process becomes quite cyclical. The more anxious we are, the more we worry. The more we worry, the more anxious we become.

This is where exercise can help break the cycle. By going for a walk or jog and looking at the scenery or taking part in a workout at the gym, our minds are automatically drawn away from our troubling thoughts as we concentrate on completing our workout. This time-out from worry has been scientifically shown to reduce feelings of anxiety.

It only stands to reason that if both the thermogenic and distraction explanations make sense by themselves, a combination of the two viewpoints would make even more sense. The most likely result of exercise is that it results in *both* body warming *and* distraction. When these two effects are combined, the result is reduced anxiety in the exerciser.

Now that we have shown exercise to have great potential for reducing anxiety in the participant and provided possible explanations for its beneficial effects, it is important to consider how exercise can be used most effectively. The following sections will tell you which exercises are best, as well as how hard, how long, and how often you must exercise to obtain the best results.

What Exercises Are Best?

If you have made the choice to try exercise in your fight against daily stressors and anxiety, it is important to determine if some exercises are more effective than others. So far, researchers have utilized a wide variety of exercises in an attempt to answer this important question. The most notable result is that several different types of exercise appear to be effective. Let's look at those that have the most potential for combating stress and anxiety.

Exercise Guideline 4.1
Running, walking, cycling, and swimming are the physical activities that have been found to be most often associated with reduced anxiety in the participant. It is interesting to note that all of these activities are rhythmic in nature and involve the use of large muscle groups.

Several studies have attempted to compare the effects of different types of exercise on anxiety, to see if one is better than the other. One experiment compared walking and jogging in terms of their potential to reduce anxiety in the participant. The results of this study indicated that both exercises resulted in significant improvement, and both appeared equally effective.

In another study,[3] 38 healthy male adults were divided into three groups. Groups 1 and 2 used jogging and weight lifting as their respective exercises, while the third group performed no exercise at all. At the conclusion of the experiment, both exercise groups experienced reduced anxiety, and both exercises were equally effective.

And finally, one large experiment[4] compared yoga, fencing, weight lifting, swimming, and jogging in terms of their potential to reduce anxiety. In this particular study, yoga produced the best results. All other exercises, however, appeared equal in their anxiety-reducing effects. While this would tend to indicate that yoga is a superior exercise for fighting anxiety, a word of caution is in order. So far, only one study has used yoga as the exercise of choice. For this reason, the reader should consider choosing another type of exercise that has consistently shown improvements across a wide range of studies. When more research is conducted, yoga may well prove to be an effective exercise for fighting anxiety.

Since several different types of exercise appear effective in fighting anxiety, the best solution is to go back to Exercise Guideline 4.1 and pick the one you like best. Once you have done this, turn to chapter 5 and read about your exercise of choice. This will provide you with information regarding the equipment you will need to get started, technical advice, helpful hints, and even a sample beginner's program. But before you start, remember to read the section at the beginning of chapter 5 to determine if exercise is safe for you.

How Often Should I Exercise?

Now that you have chosen the exercise that has the most appeal, it is important to determine just how often you must exercise to obtain the desired improvements. You will recall that earlier in this chapter we distinguished between state and trait anxiety. State anxiety represents "right now" types of feelings, whereas trait anxiety indicates a tendency to be anxious across a wide range of situations and over a prolonged period of time. This distinction is important and will help you in deciding how often you should exercise to obtain the desired improvements. Consider the following example. In this case, exercise is used in a unique way.

Fiona's Fear

Most of the time, Fiona was a relaxed and worry-free individual. The major exception occurred in the week immediately preceding her regular visit to the dentist's office. At this time, she would find herself becoming increasingly more nervous right up until the day of the appointment. By the time the morning of the checkup rolled around, Fiona was almost frantic. She told herself that she was being silly and had nothing to worry about, but this didn't seem to help. In fact, on the day of her last scheduled appointment, Fiona phoned the dental office and told them she had to cancel, since she was feeling ill. When asked when she wanted to rebook, she merely said that she would have to check her schedule and get back to them. After this last bout of anxiety on dentist day, Fiona seriously questioned whether she would be able to force herself to call for an appointment. For this reason, she arranged to see her family physician and during her visit requested a small number of Valium pills. Her doctor would not go along with this request and told her she should consider talking to a professional who dealt with this kind of problem. Unable to admit that her problems were that severe, Fiona mustered up the courage to schedule another appointment at the dental office. Unfortunately, when the dreaded day rolled around, the same symptoms appeared all over again. Two hours before her appointment, she picked up the phone, entered the first three numbers, then put the phone back on the cradle. Feeling she had to get out of the house, Fiona grabbed her jacket and started walking along a bike path near her apartment. Much to her surprise, after about 10 minutes of walking, Fiona found herself starting to relax and not worry so much about the dentist. In fact, by the time she returned to her apartment, her extreme anxiety was almost gone. At this point, Fiona got in her car, went to her appointment, and vowed to do exactly the same thing before her next visit to the dentist.

If you feel your symptoms most closely resemble state anxiety, and you don't feel you are an anxious person in general, then the following guideline will be appropriate for you.

Exercise Guideline 4.2

For state anxiety, or anxiety that has a definite cause, such as an upcoming job interview or a first date, a single bout of exercise may be all you need to feel less anxious. This reduction in state anxiety is temporary and usually lasts only four to six hours following participation in the physical activity.

In other words, exercise can be used effectively as a Band-Aid approach to reducing anxiety. In fact, there is every reason to believe that exercise may prove as effective as a minor tranquilizer for reducing situational anxiety. This is an important fact to keep in mind, since exercise is basically free, will not lead to addiction, and is not associated with the usual undesirable side effects.

Although exercise has just been portrayed as a quick fix for anxiety, and there is every reason to believe that it is, you will achieve your best results if you incorporate exercise into your lifestyle. When this is done, you will become more resistant to stress, will lower your baseline anxiety, and will reap the physical benefits as well. If this is your goal, research can once again provide an indication of how often you should exercise to produce the best and most lasting results.

Exercise Guideline 4.3
Exercise must be performed a minimum of three times per week to reduce a participant's trait anxiety. However, if you choose a lower-intensity physical activity, such as walking, it is possible to exercise four or even five times per week without any risk of overuse injuries.

If you choose a more intense type of workout, try to limit your participation to three times per week. Some research indicates that more frequent involvement may actually increase your trait anxiety. A possible explanation for this finding is that if vigorous exercise is performed too frequently, it may actually become a stressor itself. In this case, exercise just becomes too much work and too taxing on the body and the mind. When this happens, the physical activity loses its potential to lower your levels of stress and anxiety.

How Hard Should I Exercise?

You will be happy to hear that it is not necessary to exercise until exhaustion to receive the positive benefits. Early researchers in this area believed that exercise had to be performed at a moderate to high level of intensity in order to reduce anxiety. Recent research, however, has shown this original position to be incorrect. This is indeed good news to most of us who want to start an exercise program.

Exercise Guideline 4.4
It is not necessary to exercise at high intensity in order to produce significant improvements in anxiety. In fact, both moderate- and even low-intensity exercises appear every bit as effective as the more strenuous activities. If you are beginning an exercise program, it is a good idea to start exercising at a mild-intensity level, then work your way up to more strenuous workouts if you want to increase your overall level of fitness.

In support of this recent guideline, one research study[5] found that slow walking at a comfortable pace has also produced improvements in anxiety. The findings from this study provide reasonable proof that exercise does not have to be overly tiring to produce the desired benefits. Even a nice relaxing walk after supper has the potential to reduce our overall levels of anxiety.

How Long Should I Exercise?

Once again, the extensive research that has been completed provides us with more good news. It now appears that it is not necessary to exercise for long periods to experience positive benefits. This means that almost everyone can find the time to exercise.

Exercise Guideline 4.5

Exercise sessions should last at least 15 to 20 minutes in order to produce noticeable reductions in anxiety. Although some research reports even shorter exercise durations have been effective, not enough studies have been done to suggest reducing this time frame.

Obviously, if you pick walking as your exercise of choice, you may want to work your way up to longer exercise durations. This is an individual choice. If all the exercise time you can fit into your schedule is 15 to 20 minutes, by all means take that short stroll on your lunch hour or after supper. However, if you want to combine your exercise sessions with longer periods of time-out, take that walk along the river or bike path and enjoy the view. You will be surprised to see how fast the time goes by when your exercise session is surrounded by pleasant scenery.

On the other hand, if you pick a more intense type of physical activity, such as jogging or aerobic dance, it is a good idea to restrict your exercise sessions to the shorter time period. If you still feel the need to exercise longer, remember to build up gradually to a longer session.

How Soon Will I See Improvement?

As you have already seen in an earlier section, it is possible to experience noticeable reductions in anxiety with a single bout of exercise. If you wish to use exercise in this manner, you would exercise only when you are feeling anxious. Although there is nothing wrong with this approach, you will obviously obtain longer-lasting benefits if exercise becomes a part of your regular routine. Only an ongoing exercise program has the ability to lower your overall level of trait anxiety and make you more resistant to stress.

> ### *Exercise Guideline 4.6*
> **Exercise programs must be performed for a minimum of nine weeks to result in significant improvements in trait anxiety. In reality, it is likely that exercise will have to become part of your regular lifestyle if you wish to continue experiencing the beneficial effects.**

Support for this exercise guideline is provided by a very well-designed study,[6] in which 100 male and female adults were categorized into one of five jogging patterns. The categories were based on the participant's length of commitment to jogging. The advanced jogging group included individuals who had jogged for more than one year. An intermediate jogging group had jogged for between four months and one year. A beginner's group reported that they had jogged for two weeks to four months. A fourth group included those individuals who had started a jogging program, but had dropped out. A final group was represented by nonexercisers.

The results of this study showed that all jogging groups experienced lower levels of trait anxiety than did nonjoggers. Another important finding was that the advanced joggers experienced significantly lower levels of trait anxiety than did participants in any of the other groups. This led to the obvious conclusion that if physical activity is to be effective, individuals must persist in their programs over time.

Some Final Helpful Hints

Pick an exercise that you personally find appealing.
It is important that the physical activity you choose be one that seems as if it would be fun for you to do on a regular basis. If you simply join an exercise class because it is available, or choose an activity for the sake of convenience, you may find that it will not give you the desired benefits. Remember, it is *your* anxiety that you are trying to reduce, so it should be *your* choice of activity to perform. For example, if you join an aerobic dance class, but would really rather dance alone in the privacy of your house, you may find that these forced conditions actually increase your anxiety. For this reason, it is important to match the exercise to your personal preferences.

Think relaxing thoughts while you exercise.

Earlier in this chapter, you read how exercise can reduce anxiety by providing a form of distraction, or time-out. For exercise to be effective in this regard, it is important that you not dwell on those troubling thoughts that are causing your anxiety in the first place. In other words, if you focus on worrisome thoughts while exercising, it is unlikely that the physical activity can help lower anxiety. Its positive effects will be negated by your anxious thought content. A far better approach is to think pleasant thoughts, such as planning an enjoyable vacation or recalling a relaxing time on the beach.

Learn to listen to your body for stress signals.

Since exercise can be used as a Band-Aid approach to situational anxiety, it is important for you to learn to recognize when you are becoming stressed out. Take another look at the Anxiety Checklist presented earlier in this chapter, and learn to recognize these symptoms. Once you do, the solution is as simple as going for a walk or jog to immediately lower these feelings of anxiety. After a tough morning at work or a confrontation with the boss, try to get out for a brief walk during your lunchtime or coffee break. This simple procedure can help immensely, but remember, you have to learn to recognize the signs.

Don't get carried away with your exercise program.

Many people, once they start an exercise program, come to adopt a "more is better" philosophy. They believe that if three exercise sessions per week are good, then six or seven sessions will be that much better. Unfortunately, this is not the case. Unless you are exercising for reasons other than health (e.g., competitive sports or training for a road race), these added exercise sessions can actually increase your overall level of anxiety. The extra exercise sessions soon come to be seen as just another stressor in your already eventful life. For this reason, try to stick to the exercise guideline presented earlier in this chapter.

Be flexible if you don't gain the desired benefits.

If, after a few weeks into your new exercise program, you are not noticing the sought-after improvements, you may need to make some adjustments. It obviously makes no sense continuing to stick with the same program if it is definitely not working. If this happens to you, there are two solutions you should consider. The first logical approach is to try a different exercise. It may just be that this exercise is not for you. Go back to chapter 5 and reread the section on popular exercises that can improve your mental health. Then pick an alternate activity, and give it a try for a few weeks. This is often all it takes to start noticing the benefits you originally sought. Another approach is to make your original workout a little more strenuous. This does not mean that the exercise should be very difficult, but rather that you pick up your pace just a bit. This may result in more body warming and therefore more of a relaxing effect.

Exercise to your favorite music.

Many people find it much more relaxing if they listen to some of their favorite music when they exercise. This can be done by carrying a Walkman or working out in your own home where you can control what music is played. Two different types of music have great potential. Music such as "easy listening" or "instrumental favorites" is relaxing for some individuals. Others like the music to be more lively and therefore more distracting from their worries. The important thing to remember is to experiment and find the type of music that is best for you. There is no one magical type of tune that is more effective than others. It is entirely a matter of personal choice.

Try some variety in your workouts.

If you do the same exercise all the time, it is only natural that you will eventually experience some boredom with your workouts. For this reason, substitute an occasional different type of physical activity into your program. This can be done by actually planning the activity or spontaneously making the substitution. In the latter case, let's say you have chosen swimming as your exercise. On the day of your scheduled workout, you notice that the weather is exceptionally pleasant and the leaves are changing color. In situations such as this one, don't hesitate to go for a nice walk and take in the sights. Variety in your workouts can go a long way in helping you reduce your overall levels of anxiety.

Review chapters 5 and 6 before starting your program.

Remember to read the section in chapter 5 that helps you determine if exercise is safe. If you need more information on your choice of activity, read the rest of the chapter. Then take the time to read chapter 6, since this chapter will provide you with all the information you need to help you stick to your exercise program.

Looking Back

In chapter 4, you read how stress is a big part of our lives. Although we can't avoid much of this stress, the manner in which we deal with it, or interpret it, is more within our control. In this chapter, you learned how exercise has the potential to increase your resistance to daily stressors. This, in turn, can help prevent many of the problems associated with anxiety. To get a feel for your own anxiety level, you were asked to complete the Anxiety Checklist. Several traditional treatments for anxiety were presented, and you learned of the effectiveness of cognitive therapy and medication. At this point, you were provided with the exercise treatment option. A discussion of how exercise fights anxiety suggested that a combination of body warming and distraction provided the best explanation for the beneficial effects. You were then told how any exercise that is rhythmic in nature and involves the large muscle groups (e.g., running, walking, cycling, swimming) produced the best anxiety-reducing effects. You should also exercise at least three times per week for 15 to 20 minutes per session at a mild- or moderate-intensity level. A minimum of nine weeks was shown to be required for lasting results, although an individual exercise session can also be used as a Band-Aid approach.

Note

1. Stephens, T. (1988). Physical and mental health in the United States and Canada: Evidence from four population surveys. *Preventive Medicine, 17*, 35–47.

2. Crocker, P.R., & Grozelle, C. (1991). Reducing induced state anxiety: Effects of acute aerobic exercise and autogenic relaxation. *The Journal of Sports Medicine and Physical Fitness, 31*, 277–282.

3. Sinyor, D., Golden, M., Steinert, Y., & Seraganian, P. (1986). Experimental manipulation of aerobic fitness and the response to psychosocial stress: Heart rate and self-report measures. *Psychosomatic Medicine, 45*, 324–337.

4. Berger, B.G., & Owen, D.R. (1988). Stress reduction and mood enhancement in four exercise modes: Swimming, body conditioning, hatha yoga, and fencing. *Research Quarterly, 59*, 145–159.

5. Sexton, H., Maere, A., & Dahl, N. (1989). Exercise intensity and reduction in neurotic symptoms: A controlled study. *Acta-Psychiatrica-Scandinavia, 80*, 231–235.

6. Nouri, S., & Beer, J. (1989). Relations of moderate physical exercise to scores on hostility, aggression, and trait anxiety. *Perceptual and Motor Skills, 68*, 1191–1194.

CHAPTER 5

POPULAR EXERCISES THAT WILL IMPROVE YOUR MENTAL HEALTH

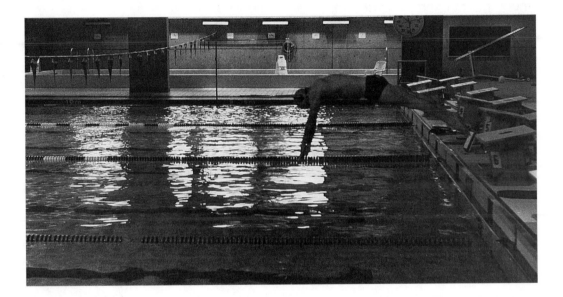

Just like with most things in life, there is a right way and a wrong way to exercise. Now that you have seen some of the psychological benefits that can result from regular participation in an exercise program, it is time to turn our attention to the exercises themselves.

In this chapter, you will
✓ learn if exercise is safe for you personally.
✓ be exposed to a variety of exercises that can improve your mental health.
✓ be in the position to choose the type of exercise you want to try.
✓ learn what equipment you need to start your program.
✓ get basic instruction in the technical aspects of your exercise of choice.
✓ be provided with a sample beginner's program to get you started.

Before You Begin

Before you do anything else, it is absolutely essential that you determine if exercise is safe for you. The best ways to do this are the standard medical examination and the completion of a standardized checklist. Let's look at each of these in turn.

Is a Medical Examination Necessary?

There is no simple answer to this question. However, some guidelines will help you determine if you should have a medical examination before commencing an exercise program.

The general rule is that a complete medical examination *and* a diagnostic exercise test should be performed on males over 40 years of age and females over 50 years of age before starting a *vigorous* exercise program. This same rule applies even if the would-be participant is a seemingly healthy individual. Remember, we are talking about a vigorous, or high-intensity, exercise program. If you are beginning a mild- or moderate-intensity regimen, then these procedures are not necessary.

For all individuals who have been determined to be at higher coronary risk (e.g., physically inactive people, smokers, people with hypertension or high cholesterol), a maximal exercise test performed by a physician is required.

Finally, it has been determined that healthy individuals of any age can be effectively screened by means of validated questions, such as those presented in the following Personal Health Checklist, provided that the questions are answered accurately and honestly. If you have any reason to believe that exercise may not be safe for you, *or* if you just feel you would like the peace of mind associated with a medical examination, then by all means have one performed. The key point is to play it safe.

Another of the easiest and most accepted ways of learning about the safety of exercise is by simply answering several important questions. Read through the following checklist and place a check mark (✓) beside any question that you would answer "Yes." Remember, it is essential that you answer these questions honestly. There are no right or wrong answers, just answers that apply to you as an individual.

A PERSONAL HEALTH CHECKLIST

1. Has your doctor ever told you that you have a heart condition *and* should do only those exercises that are prescribed by a doctor?   _____

2. Do you feel pain in your chest when you do physical activity?   _____

3. In the past month, have you had any chest pain when you were not doing physical activity?   _____

4. Do you ever lose your balance because of dizziness, *or* do you ever faint?   _____

5. Do you have any bone or joint problem that could be made worse by exercise?   _____

6. Is your doctor currently prescribing drugs (e.g., water pills) for your blood pressure or heart condition?   _____

7. Do you know of *any other reason* why you should not exercise?   _____

If you checked "Yes" to one or more of the questions on the checklist, you should talk to your doctor, either by phone or in person, *before* you take any form of fitness appraisal and *before* you start your exercise program. Tell your doctor about the questions to which you answered "Yes." In many cases, you may be able to do any activity you want, provided you start slowly and build up gradually. In other cases, and depending on your answers to the questions, it may be necessary to restrict your physical activities to those that are safe for you. Consult your doctor about the types of exercise you would like to perform, *and then take his or her advice.*

If you honestly answered "No" to all of the questions, you can be reasonably sure that you can start an exercise program. You may, however, want to have a fitness appraisal done by an expert to provide additional guidance in selecting an activity.

The Exercises

Now that you have taken the necessary precautions to determine if exercise is safe, let's turn our attention to the physical activities themselves. The remainder of this chapter will focus on a variety of popular exercises that have the potential to improve your mental health. Take a few minutes and read through these descriptions. Then pick the activity that has the most appeal to you. By following the recommendations for your activity of choice, you are ensuring a positive exercise experience. Before you do this, read the following case, which depicts an individual who started an exercise program without weighing the options.

Amy's Alternative

Looking in the mirror, Amy decided that the time had finally come to get back in shape. Although she hadn't gained too much weight, it was obvious that some muscle toning and firming up were in order. Armed with this new resolve, Amy promised herself that she would start a regular exercise program within the week. Because she had been an avid swimmer many years before, this seemed like the right exercise to adopt. Swimming posed no problem, since a community pool was available where she could pay a small fee each visit. No membership was required. Although the first few times in the pool were invigorating, Amy found that she quickly became bored with this activity. This surprised her since she had swum regularly for several years. Now, however, swimming just didn't seem as much fun. For this reason, Amy looked through the calendar of activities put out by the city recreation department. She noticed a large number of offerings for low-impact aerobics. In fact, open classes were offered every noon hour at a local recreation facility. Amy decided to give this activity a try the following week. In her very first session, she knew that she had found her activity. The instructor was fun, the music was lively, and it was great to have other people around. After several weeks, Amy and a few other exercisers started going out for coffee after the exercise sessions. This added social dimension turned out to be a real plus for Amy and kept her coming back.

To ensure that you don't repeat Amy's mistake, read through the following exercises and pick the one that is best for you.

Walking

Walking represents the most natural form of physical activity known to people. For this reason, we are ideally suited for this type of exercise. In its simplest form, walking is merely a matter of putting one foot in front of the other — something that most of us have mastered by one year of age. Walking has become a popular form of exercise because it can be done anywhere at any time. Choosing walking as your preferred type of exercise has several additional advantages:

- It doesn't require much time or effort to learn the proper technique.
- It doesn't cost much to get started.

- There is a low injury rate.
- You can actually become more physically fit, as long as you walk long enough, fast enough, and often enough.
- If you travel, your walking program travels with you.
- You can enjoy your favorite music by taking along a Walkman — it won't fall off as often as it might with other exercises.
- Walking is a weight-bearing activity that can help prevent osteoporosis.

Recommended Equipment

The equipment you need to start a walking program is simple: good shoes and comfortable clothing. Let's take a brief look at what you need from each of these two categories.

Walking shoes. If you are strapped for cash, almost any low-heeled shoe can be used to start a walking program. If at all possible, however, invest in a good pair of walking shoes. This will not only make the activity more enjoyable, but will also help you avoid foot, ankle, knee, hip, and lower back problems. As a bonus, good shoes will prevent the development of nagging problems, such as blisters, calluses, or "hot spots."

When shopping for this important piece of equipment, remember that walking shoes are different from running shoes. In fact, even the best running shoes are inappropriate for a walking program. This is because walking shoes need to be more flexible, since you bend your feet more when you walk and push off harder from your toes. Also, because your heels bear most of your weight when you walk, you need a good stable *heel counter.* This is the part of the shoe that wraps around your heel to keep your foot in place.

If you decide to go shopping for a pair of walking shoes, remember to pay special attention to the following details:

- If you have an old pair of walking shoes, or even regular shoes that are well-worn, take these along to show the salesclerk. The old shoes can show wear patterns and help identify your special needs.
- Take along a pair of sweat socks that are the same type you will be wearing when you exercise. This will allow you to get a better fit when you buy your shoes.
- Remember to try on *both* the left and right shoes. Then walk on a hard floor surface that does not have carpeting.
- Pay special attention to pressure areas and any slipping. These could eventually cause troublesome blisters.
- Don't rush into the purchase. Take your time so that your feet will have a chance to settle into the shoes.

Appropriate clothing. Once again, if money is an issue, almost any type of clothing will do the trick. You will enjoy your activity much more, however, if you follow a few basic principles. Perhaps the most important characteristic is how comfortable the clothing feels. Most people tend to prefer loose-fitting clothes that allow for greater freedom of motion.

Another important factor to consider is the climate in which you live. In hot weather, light, breathable clothes made of fabrics such as cotton will prove most comfortable. In contrast, in cold temperatures it is always advisable to wear several layers of thin clothing for maximum warmth. If you don't mind a little extra expense, consider investing in a polypropylene top. It is also necessary to keep your head and hands warm, since a good deal of body heat is lost from these areas.

The Proper Walking Technique

To get the most out of your walking program, you need to pay special attention to your form. The most common mistake that walkers make is bending forward too much at the waist. This almost always leads to the development of problems in your lower back, hips, and neck. While you shouldn't force yourself to be ramrod straight, your posture should be "naturally tall." Try to relax your shoulders, widen your chest, and pull your stomach muscles gently inward. Keep your head and chin up, and focus your attention straight ahead. Think in terms of "walking proud" rather than "walking embarrassed."

Most experts believe that it is important to relax your hands while keeping them gently cupped. Your arms should swing gently past your hips. At the uppermost position, your hands should be approximately level with your breast bone. On the downswing, your hands should gently brush your hips.

And finally, it is important that you learn to "roll." Always try to land on your heels, then roll your feet forward, pushing off with your toes.

If you are thinking that all of this sounds pretty complicated, don't despair. Most people walk with pretty good form already. We just need a little fine-tuning from time to time. For this reason, it is always a good idea to take ourselves through a head-to-toe checklist every once in a while.

A Sample Program for Beginners

The following program is intended for those individuals who are *starting* a walking program. In most cases, you will be walking at a 20 to 30 minute-per-mile pace.

Week	Day 1	Day 2	Day 3	Day 4	Day 5	Day 6	Day 7
1	20			20			20
2	20			25			20
3	20		20		20		20
4	20		25		20		30
5	20		25		25		30
6	20	25		20	25		20
7	20	25		20	25		25
8	25	25		25	20		30
9	25	25		30	25		30

Note: All daily totals are in minutes of walking.

In Weeks 10 through 12, feel free to increase your total time spent walking in some or all of the sessions. If you take this approach, remember to make your increases gradual, just like in the earlier weeks.

Some Final Hints

Think safety.

If you walk alone, carry identification. It is also important to remain aware of what is going on around you. Avoid deserted routes if possible. It is always safer to walk in a public place. And finally, if you walk at night, remember to wear reflective clothing.

Walk at a good pace.

Perhaps a good guideline is to walk as fast as you comfortably can. Don't overdo it, but a somewhat faster walking pace will burn more calories and give you greater fitness gains.

Sneak in a walk whenever possible.

Try to leave your car at home and walk to the variety store. You can also start parking your car at the outside perimeter of the parking lot, then walk to the mall entrance from there. All of these little extras add up over time. Recent evidence suggests "accumulated exercise" during the day can pay big dividends.

Consider the use of hand weights.

Many experts now have come to realize the value of hand and leg weights. These can speed up the fitness process. They are relatively inexpensive and can be purchased in most department stores.

Enjoy yourself.

Do whatever it takes to have fun walking. Remember, the more you enjoy it, the easier it will be to stick with your program.

If you get sore, take some time off.

If you find your muscles are hurting, take the next day or two off. You may also want to consider Deep Cold applications. This product is available over the counter at most drug stores.

Jogging

Like walking, jogging is a relatively simple activity that you can take with you anywhere you travel. You don't need a bagful of equipment, a swimming pool, or a rack on the roof of your car. You simply put on your running gear, open the door, and go. Jogging has become a popular form of exercise since it offers several distinct advantages for the participant:

- It doesn't require much learning, since it is an activity we developed in childhood.
- Running gear is relatively inexpensive.
- Jogging is an excellent exercise for the heart and lungs.
- You can experience the physical and mental benefits in a relatively short period of time.
- You can do it almost anywhere.

Although these advantages make jogging look like a attractive exercise, it is certainly not for everyone. Some runners tend to have frequent and ongoing injuries. Many of these individuals probably have lower backs, hips, knees, and ankles that simply cannot take all the pounding. If you are not built to run, don't try to force this activity on yourself. You can experience all of the physical and mental benefits with the other exercises described in this chapter.

Recommended Equipment

Although it is entirely possible to spend hundreds of dollars on fancy running gear, the only essential equipment is a good pair of running shoes. Although running shoe prices vary greatly, you should expect to pay a minimum of $40 to $50 a pair. Don't be fooled by the salesperson who tells you that you must spend $100 or more to avoid injuries. In fact, an interesting anecdote concerns the podiatrist who was asked the difference between a $60 shoe and a $100 shoe. His simple answer was "about $40."

Even so, it is always a good idea to shop at a running shoe store that is staffed by runners. Don't be afraid to ask if the salesperson has experience running. These individuals will help you decide the type of shoe that is best for you. They will take important factors into consideration, such as your running goals, shape of your foot, weight, and even any special problems you may have, such as bad knees or lower back pain that may require special consideration.

Your shoes should feel comfortable from the moment you try them on. Don't fall for the old sales pitch that tells you they need to be broken in before they will fit well and feel comfortable.

The two features you should look for in a running shoe are flexibility and a good heel counter. To determine if a shoe has proper flexibility, hold it at both ends, and bend it. The shoe should bend right at the ball of the foot. This will provide your feet with the needed range of motion while jogging. The second key feature of a running shoe is the same as what was required in a good walking shoe — a stable heel counter. This will prevent your foot's slipping around, movement that can cause a variety of joint injuries.

And finally, you will want to have some comfortable clothing for your run. This needn't be expensive — an old sweatsuit will do the trick. If you want a trendier look, you can always opt for the fancy warm-ups, or even the Spandex clothing. Decisions of this nature are obviously a matter of personal choice and finance.

The Proper Jogging Technique

Almost everyone has a jogging style that is somewhat unique. This is because our actual technique is determined to a large extent by our physical makeup. Height, weight, limb length, and joint flexibility are just some of the individual differences that produce our personal jogging styles. For this reason, it is important not to worry too much about form at this point. Instead, just try to enjoy yourself and do what comes naturally. You will find the activity less tiring if you remember to relax your shoulders and arms, then let your arms swing loosely. It is also recommended that you not run with clenched fists. When we tense all of these muscles, running with a smooth gait becomes difficult. Tension also makes the activity more tiring and less enjoyable.

Once you have been jogging for a while, start to pay a bit more attention to your posture. Keep your head up and your eyes focused straight ahead. It is also a good idea to avoid leaning too far forward at the hips. When people jog with their eyes glued to the ground in front of them and with their body bent over at the hips, they are setting themselves up for pain and discomfort in the neck, upper back, lower back, and hips. So remember to jog relaxed, jog tall, and look at a point approximately 30 feet in front of you. Utilizing this proper technique will allow you to get more enjoyment out of this excellent activity.

A Sample Program for Beginners

The following sample program is intended for people who are new to the jogging scene. Because jogging is a relatively strenuous activity, it is important to build up slowly. For this reason, you will notice that the first few weeks are devoted solely to walking. The next step involves a combination of walking and jogging. Perhaps the best guideline when you enter this phase is to jog only as much as you can comfortably: then return to walking until you feel able to jog again. Repeat this process for your allotted duration as indicated in the sample program. When you reach the final phase, you have "graduated" — all jogging and no walking!

Week	Day 1	Day 2	Day 3	Day 4	Day 5	Day 6	Day 7
1	W/15		W/15		W/15		
2	W/15		W/15		W/15		
3	W/15		W/15		W/15		
4	WJ/15		WJ/15		WJ/15		
5	WJ/15		WJ/15		WJ/15		
6	WJ/15		WJ/15		WJ/15		
7	J/15		WJ/15		J/15		
8	J/15		WJ/15		J/15		
9	J/15		J/15		J/15		

Note: All daily totals are in minutes.
W=Walk, J=Jog

After the conclusion of Week 9, you can maintain this schedule indefinitely. It will give you all the exercise you really need. If you want to increase your jogging time to 20-minute sessions, feel free to do so. Jogging more than 15–20 minutes three times per week is not necessary unless you have taken up jogging for reasons other than improved physical and mental health.

Some Final Hints

Enjoy your exercise.

It is essential that you enjoy your exercise experience. You are not likely to stick with a jogging program if it makes you miserable. The best way to learn to enjoy jogging is to start slowly. Don't push yourself too hard or too fast, or you will find yourself tempted to skip exercise sessions. Remind yourself that you do not gain any additional benefit from tuckering yourself out.

Use a walk/jog transition technique.

Remember to ease into your program by alternating periods of walking with periods of jogging. (See sample program, Week 4.) Two minutes walking and one minute jogging is a good place to start once you have progressed beyond the "walking only" break-in period. Gradually increase your jogging intervals until you are able to jog continuously for 15 to 20 minutes.

Run economically.

Try not to bounce or overstride. Relax the muscles in your arms and upper body, and you will find the activity far less tiring.

Watch out for motorists.

If you must run on the road, make sure you follow these safety guidelines.

Run facing the traffic, and make sure you are visible. If you jog at night, make sure you wear reflective clothing.

Swimming

Swimming has been called one of the most complete forms of exercise. In fact, many health professionals and almost all swimmers consider swimming to be the best exercise, period. While this may or may not be true, a good case can be made for choosing this type of exercise. The major advantages of swimming include the following points:

- Swimming is a zero-impact exercise. There is no pounding on your joints.
- You have a great aerobic workout that uses your whole body.
- Swimming stretches the major muscle groups, thereby improving flexibility.
- Depending on your location and choice of facilities, swimming represents a relatively inexpensive form of exercise.
- Swimming is great for people who are pregnant or overweight, as well as for individuals who want to keep exercising when they are injured from another activity.

Recommended Equipment

In addition to a pool or body of water that is preferably staffed by a lifeguard, all you really need (from a legal perspective) is a swimsuit. If you swim in a chlorinated pool or a body of salt water, goggles and a swim cap are recommended. The goggles will prevent eye irritation, while the cap will protect your hair from the harsh chemicals.

Other items of equipment you may wish to consider include hand paddles, rubber swimming fins, and a kickboard. Some individuals like to use earplugs and nose clips. These are strictly a matter of individual preference.

The Proper Swimming Technique

It is almost impossible to learn to swim by reading a book. Your best bet is to enroll in swimming lessons or to recruit a friend who is an experienced swimmer. It is important that you receive constant feedback concerning your stroke. More than any other exercise, swimming relies on technique. It will take time to develop the specific swimming style that will allow you to swim efficiently and enjoyably.

The few technical points that follow refer to the freestyle stroke. Most people prefer this style because it allows them to go faster. If you prefer a different stroke, no problem. You can obtain a good enough workout from any type of swimming.

In performing the freestyle, there are a few technical points you should keep in mind. First, make sure you don't "cut your strokes short." Try to reach out as far as you can, then pull all the way through the water so that your hand brushes your thigh. This will require fewer strokes to swim the same distance.

A second important point is to keep your elbow higher than any other part of your arm or hand during the entire stroke. This technical point will provide you with more power from your stroke. In addition, as your hand enters the water in front of you, remember to lead with your thumb, then relax your hand, and keep your fingers slightly apart (not tightly clenched).

Finally, make sure you kick up and down from your hips, not your knees. Try not to kick too deeply or allow your feet to break the water's surface. This will provide you with the maximum thrust, making you go faster with less effort.

A Sample Program for Beginners

The following program is intended for people who know how to swim, but have not participated in this activity for months or even years. Because swimming is a relatively intense exercise, especially for individuals who do not swim regularly, it is important to start slowly. For this reason, the first few weeks of the beginner's program are flexible and include lots of rest time. Use your swim and rest (S/R) time guidelines as you see fit.

Start by seeing how long you can swim comfortably; then rest until you can repeat the process. Don't worry about how far or how long you can initially swim without a rest. This will improve with time. Remember, you can keep moving even during rest periods by walking around slowly in shallow water. As you grow more comfortable with this exercise, try to increase the amount of time you swim and decrease the amount of time you rest.

Week	Day 1	Day 2	Day 3	Day 4	Day 5	Day 6	Day 7
1	SR/5		SR/5		SR/5		
2	SR/5		SR/10		SR/5		
3	SR/10		SR/5		SR/10		
4	SR/10		SR/10		SR/10		
5	SR/10		SR/15		SR/10		
6	SR/15		SR/10		SR/15		
7	SR/15		SR/15		SR/15		
8	SR/20		SR/15		SR/20		
9	SR/20		SR/20		SR/20		

Note: All daily totals are in minutes. Gradually decrease the amount of rest time (R) and increase the amount of swim time (S).

After the conclusion of Week 9, you can maintain this schedule indefinitely. The important thing to remember is that you should be getting at least 15 to 20 minutes of actual swim time in your workouts.

Some Final Hints

Think safety first.

Never swim shortly after a meal, since this can cause dangerous cramping. Never swim alone, and never swim in open water unless you are experienced *and* have an equally experienced friend with you.

Take a refresher course.

Swimming relies on technique more than any of the other exercises discussed in this chapter. For this reason, it is probably a good idea to take a few lessons as a refresher course. This way, you won't waste so much time splashing around instead of moving forward.

Consider using swimming aids.

Following from the preceding hint, you might want to consider investing in a pair of swimming (speed) fins. This will make the exercise more enjoyable initially and allow you to move fast enough to get a good workout.

Consider alternative water exercises.

If swimming starts to become too boring for you, consider water running or water aerobics. Both of these options will provide you with all the same advantages as swimming.

Cycling

Learning to ride a bicycle is relatively simple. Most of us master this skill early in childhood. But if you want to become a good cyclist, then be prepared to work hard on your technique. The choice is yours, so ask yourself if you want something out of this exercise in addition to the physical and mental benefits. In either case, a good argument can be made for choosing this exercise mode. The most frequently mentioned advantages would include the following:

- Cycling is a perfect choice for people who can't take the continuous pounding on the joints caused by jogging. In fact, many cyclists are ex-joggers.
- Cycling is an excellent way to lose weight. Even cycling at 12 m.p.h., a relatively slow pace, burns almost as many calories as jogging.
- It is easy to see your progress. Even a beginning cyclist can build up to a 20-mile ride quite easily.
- Cycling is not as boring as some of the other types of exercise. Because you can vary your cycling routes, you are continually seeing new scenery.

Recommended Equipment

No matter how you look at it, cycling requires a lot of equipment. Unlike several of the other exercises, you can't just buy a bike and get the rest of the gear later. In this section, we will look at what equipment is essential and suggest a few extras you may want to add later.

Buying your bike. If you haven't been involved in the purchase of a bike since your school years, be prepared for a shock. Regardless of whether you buy a mountain bike or a road bike, you should be prepared to spend a minimum of $400 to $500. In fact, some bikes go for as high as $3,000, if you want state-of-the-art equipment. For the most part, however, the $400 to $500 range is a good guideline. This will get you a good bike that shouldn't break down for several years. If you are serious about cycling on a long-term basis, this price range is the bare minimum. If money is a problem, check out some garage sales and you may just be able to find a used bike at a much cheaper price.

In terms of deciding between a mountain bike and a road bike, simply ask yourself where you plan to do the majority of your cycling. If all of your exercise will be done on paved highways, then you may want a road bike. On the other hand, if you see yourself cycling on dirt roads or bike paths, then a mountain bike is the way to go. Most people tend to choose this option, with over 80% of all new purchases being mountain bikes. They are more versatile and more comfortable. Make sure you seek out a knowledgeable and trustworthy salesperson to ensure you end up with a bike that fits you.

Other recommended equipment. Aside from a bicycle, you will need a good helmet. In many localities, a helmet is required by law, as well it should be. This piece of equipment will set you back only about $30. Don't even consider starting your cycling program until you have made this purchase.

Other items you may wish to consider include cycling gloves to make your ride more comfortable and protect your hands from falls, and cycling glasses to protect your eyes from dust and gravel. Finally, a pair of padded cycling shorts and a piece of reflective clothing will make your exercise more comfortable and safe.

The Proper Cycling Technique

Cycling is an exercise that requires you to develop several new and somewhat different skills. More specifically, you need to observe a few principles of body position, gear shifting, and pedaling.

This type of physical activity can wreak havoc on your lower back, since you are in a crouched position for so long. For this reason, try to relax your upper body and keep your arms loose. Your best body position is to lean forward slightly at the waist, since this provides the most aerodynamically efficient way of slicing through the head wind.

As you cycle, remember to change your hand position regularly. This will prevent cramping or stiffness during a prolonged ride. It is also a good idea to grasp your handlebars with about the same amount of tension you would use in holding a child's hand when you cross the street. This will give you adequate control while preventing fatigue.

If you learn to shift gears properly, you will find that you can ride more efficiently and effectively. Perhaps the most common mistake inexperienced cyclists make is to use more tension than they can handle. This forces the cyclist to pedal more slowly, tire more quickly, and stop exercising sooner. The key is to select a certain cycling cadence, then shift gears as necessary to maintain this cadence. Most people experience problems because they start out in too high a gear or get caught in one when they have to climb a hill. So learn to reduce your tension. This will help you enjoy your ride.

A Sample Program for Beginners

The following sample program has been developed for novice cyclists. You will notice that there is no mention of speed or pace. This is because our primary goal is to get you to the point where you can cycle comfortably for a period of time that will allow the mental benefits to kick in.

Week	Day 1	Day 2	Day 3	Day 4	Day 5	Day 6	Day 7
1	15		15		15		
2	15		20		15		
3	20		15		20		
4	20		20		20		
5	20		25		20		
6	25		20		25		
7	25		25		25		
8	25		30		25		
9	30		25		30		

Note: All daily totals refer to the number of minutes cycled.

At the conclusion of Week 9, you have the option of maintaining this schedule or gradually increasing your time spent cycling. If you feel that Week 9 represents about as much exercise as you want to handle, don't worry. Research suggests that sessions of 20 to 30 minutes will provide you with all the mental health benefits you desire.

Some Final Hints

Follow the rules of the road, and think safety first.

Stop at all stop signs, obey all traffic signs, and remember to use those hand signals we all learned when getting our driver's license. It is also a good idea to assume the driver of a vehicle doesn't see you. This added caution could save your life.

Drink plenty of fluids.

Always take along a water bottle, and drink even before you get thirsty.

Never squeeze your brakes — especially your front brakes — with a lot of pressure.

This will cause you to go flying over the handlebars. Squeeze them gently, with uniform pressure.

Learn how to fix a flat.

If you don't learn this handy skill immediately, you could become stranded miles from home.

Know your gears.

Experiment with your gears to learn what you and your bike can and can't do. This way, when you come to a nasty hill, you won't panic and possibly tip over.

Weight Lifting

Not that long ago, working out with weights was something done almost exclusively by bodybuilders, weight lifters, or people undergoing rehabilitation from an injury. Recently, however, this activity has become a popular form of exercise for anyone interested in improving his or her level of fitness. There are several reasons for this increasing popularity:

- You can get a good, whole-body workout in a relatively short time.
- You don't have to go outside into the cold and rain to work out.
- You can see the effects of this exercise on your body within only a few weeks.
- Done properly, weight lifting can improve several aspects of fitness, including cardiovascular conditioning, strength and endurance, flexibility, and even body composition.

Recommended Equipment

You don't need a great deal of equipment to benefit from this form of exercise. In terms of clothing, all you require is a pair of sports shoes with non-marking soles and some loose-fitting clothes. A comfortable sweatsuit will do just fine. If you want to invest in a spiffy outfit, go ahead, but remember, the weights won't know the difference.

Weight lifting is usually performed with the use of weight machines or free weights. Free weights are simply bars with weight plates on each end. The long bars are called barbells, and the short bars are called dumbbells. While many experienced lifters prefer free weights, they pose several distinct disadvantages for the beginner.

The most important drawback of using free weights involves the safety factor. It is easy to lose your balance and drop the weights. And if you are performing a bench press, where you lie on your back on a bench and press the weight upwards, it is easy to be trapped under the bar if you can't muster enough strength to complete the exercise. For reasons such as these, with a special eye to the safety factor, we will focus our attention only on the use of weight machines. For most beginners to a weight-lifting program, this is the way to go.

Weight machines. Using weight machines is not as complicated as it looks. In fact, what it really boils down to is two relatively simple acts. You adjust the weight to be lifted, then either push or pull on a bar or set of handles. If the exercise you are performing is done in a sitting position, you may also have to adjust the seat position. So don't be intimidated by the appearance of these machines — they are really quite easy to use.

The basic principle behind weight machines is that the bars or handles are attached to a cable or chain, which in turn is connected to a stack of rectangular weight plates. These weight plates usually weigh between five and 20 pounds, depending on the make and model. Each plate has a hole drilled in its center, so if you want to lift 20 pounds, you simply stick a metal pin into the hole on the plate marked 20 pounds. Then, when you push or pull on the handle, the cable picks up 20 pounds.

As a general guideline, most weight machines are set up to allow you to perform six to 12 different exercises on them. These exercises have been designed to work the major muscle groups. In most gyms, pictures demonstrating each of these exercises are mounted on the wall near the machine.

Club membership or machine ownership? Obviously, this decision is a matter of personal choice and finances. The weight machines designed for home use, called multigyms, aren't quite as large or as complicated-looking as the ones you will find in health clubs. They are also nowhere near as expensive. If you shop around, you can usually find a good multigym in the $200 to $500 price range. Many people set these up in a spare bedroom, the basement, or even the garage.

On the other hand, the cost of membership in a fitness club varies tremendously. The fancier the club, the higher the fees. If you don't want all the frills, you can usually find a reasonable rate. A good guideline would be in the $150 to $300 range for a membership in a nonexclusive club. Advantages of club membership include access to cardiovascular fitness equipment, possible life insurance rebates, and the professional expertise of an instructor.

In arriving at your decision, ask yourself where you would be most likely to exercise regularly — at home or at a club. The answer to this question, in addition to your personal financial situation, should help you make up your mind.

The Proper Weight-Lifting Technique

Because a great amount of variety exists between both fitness clubs and weight machines, it is not possible to provide you with specific techniques for specific exercises. If you join a club, an instructor will be happy to familiarize you with the proper lifting techniques for that club's machines. If you buy your own multigym, it will come with an instruction booklet.

There are, however, a few general principles that you should attempt to follow. First, improvements in muscular strength and muscular endurance are accomplished by means of resistance training, and both involve a principle called *overload*. If you want to improve your strength (how much you can lift), it is best to lift larger weights a fewer number of times. If you want to improve your endurance (how often you can lift a weight), it is best to lift less weight a greater number of times. How often you lift a particular weight is usually called the number of *repetitions*.

If you want to concentrate on strength development, you should perform lifts with an amount of weight that you can repeat six times. After doing this with each of the individual exercises, you should repeat the whole process again. In weight-lifting terms, this means doing two *sets* of six *repetitions*.

If you are not as concerned with strength development, but would simply like to tone up, you should perform your lifts with an amount of weight that you can repeat 10 to 12 times. You should also repeat this process at least one time. This means you will be doing two *sets* of 10 to 12 *repetitions*.

A Sample Program for Beginners

The sample program provided here assumes that you are relatively new to this type of activity. It also makes the assumption that you are more interested in toning up than you are in bulking up. For these reasons, the program asks you to perform 10 to 12 repetitions per lift rather than six. When starting out, remember to lift weight amounts that seem "too easy" to do 12 times. This will ensure that you will not strain your muscles or be turned off by the activity. As the weeks go by, *gradually* increase the weight amounts to where you need to "work" to do all 12 repetitions.

Week	Day 1	Day 2	Day 3	Day 4	Day 5	Day 6	Day 7
1	1S/10R		1S/10R		1S/10R		
2	1S/10R		1S/10R		1S/10R		
3	1S/12R		1S/10R		1S/12R		
4	1S/12R		1S/12R		1S/12R		
5	2S/10R		1S/12R		2S/10R		
6	2S/10R		2S/10R		2S/10R		
7	2S/12R		2S/10R		2S/12R		
8	2S/12R		2S/12R		2S/12R		
9	2S/12R		2S/12R		2S/12R		

Note: All daily totals refer to the # of sets (S) and the # of repetitions (R). Weight amounts can be gradually increased as weeks progress.

At the conclusion of Week 9, you can maintain this schedule indefinitely. Feel free to add more weight for each exercise when it becomes too easy to do 12 repetitions.

Some Final Hints

Start your program easily.

This point can't be stressed enough. During your first few weeks, make certain that the amount of weight you are lifting for each of the exercises feels embarrassingly easy.

Work your entire body.

It is very important that your program exercise *all* major muscle groups, not just your arms and legs. The muscles in your trunk (stomach, sides, and upper and lower back) also need to be developed.

Check the weight stack before you lift.

Always check to see where the pin is inserted before you start your lifts. When you first start, jot down the weights that feel comfortable in a small notebook or your exercise diary (chapter 7). Refer to this list on subsequent trips to the gym and update the weight totals as needed.

Consult an instructor.

If you are unfamiliar with the weight machine or have limited knowledge about anatomy or strength training, make sure you consult the gym's trainer/instructor. This will get you started safely. After a few sessions, you will be able to train on your own.

Don't hold your breath.

Some people prefer a particular breathing pattern, such as exhaling when lifting weights and inhaling when lowering them. This is a matter of personal choice; it really isn't necessary. Just make sure that you do not hold your breath when lifting. This will limit your oxygen supply and in some cases may even cause you to faint.

Aerobic Dance and Step Aerobics

Over the past several years, *aerobics* has become popular within exercise circles. While this activity was originally the domain of women, more and more men are now enjoying the benefits of this excellent activity. There are several reasons for this growing interest:

- Aerobics requires little exercise equipment, so expenses are minimal.
- In most cases, it is performed in a group, so you can socialize when you exercise.
- It provides an excellent whole-body workout.
- It is especially good for toning your legs and buttocks.
- Because of the social element and perky music, it rarely becomes boring.
- Because of the popularity of aerobics, it is easy to find an exercise class.
- If you like to exercise alone, aerobics can be done in the privacy of your own house or apartment.

As you can see, there are several excellent reasons to choose this form of activity. However, if you have knee, back, or ankle problems, you may want to consider a different type of exercise, or at least tone down the movements to prevent aggravation in these sensitive areas.

Recommended Equipment

This form of exercise requires little equipment. All you need is a good pair of aerobics or walking shoes, with extra cushioning at the ball of the foot and reasonable ankle support. A good sports shoe salesperson can recommend several models that will fit almost anyone's budget. In addition to a good pair of shoes, you need comfortable, loose-fitting clothing. All that matters is that your exercise clothing allows for a full range of movement — split seams have caused many embarrassing moments in aerobics classes.

If you prefer step aerobics (see next section) and exercise at home, you may want to invest in a sturdy step platform. This item is not expensive. You can probably buy one for $20 to $50 at your local department store.

The Proper Aerobics Technique

Because of the nature of this exercise, it is impossible to get into technical points. This is because every instructor has a somewhat different style. It is possible, however, to give you a general idea of what to expect with this type of activity.

Originally, the term *aerobic dance* referred to one specific type of activity. Basically speaking, it involved a traditional dance-inspired exercise routine. A selection of musical recordings was played while the participants attempted to move to the music. Recently, however, aerobic dance has evolved into two separate streams — high-/low-impact aerobics and step aerobics.

High-/low-impact aerobics closely resembles the original aerobic dance, with two different styles. With low-impact, you always have one foot on the floor; there are no jumping or hopping movements. In contrast, high-impact aerobics moves at a slower pace, but you are required to hop and jump around a lot. Some instructors even combine high- and low-impact routines. In almost all cases, the exercises are performed to music, and you attempt to mimic your instructor's movements.

Step aerobics, on the other hand, involves a choreographed routine of stepping up and down on a rectangular or circular platform. This is also usually done to music while you follow your instructor's movements. If you choose this form of aerobics, make sure you never use a platform so high that your knee is higher than your hips when you step up; this can cause injuries.

A Sample Program for Beginners

The sample program here applies to either high-/low-impact aerobics or step aerobics. It also assumes that you are not a regular exerciser. For this reason, the program starts slowly. This is because this form of exercise can be hard on your body if you start out too fast. All of the numbers shown in the following schedule refer to the number of minutes the exercise is performed. If these exercise sessions are too easy for you, feel free to add more minutes. The important consideration is to start slowly and build up gradually. You will enjoy the activity more *and* avoid muscle aches and pains.

Week	Day 1	Day 2	Day 3	Day 4	Day 5	Day 6	Day 7
1	10		10		10		
2	10		15		10		
3	15		10		15		
4	15		15		15		
5	15		20		15		
6	20		15		20		
7	20		20		20		
8	20		20		20		
9	20		20		20		

Note: All daily numbers refer to the number of minutes of exercise.

At the conclusion of Week 9, you can stick with this schedule if that's what you want to do. If you want to add more exercise time, feel free to do so. And remember, if you are exercising in a class, you will have several rest breaks, so if you are enrolled in a 45-minute class, all of that time won't be spent exercising. Also, don't feel you have to do all of the exercises for the first several weeks. Do only as much as feels comfortable to you — don't worry about your exercise classmates. With time, you will be able to do everything they can. You may also wish to consider purchasing a relatively inexpensive videotape. These are especially useful if you like to exercise in the privacy of your home or have difficulty going to classes regularly.

Some Final Hints

Shop around for an instructor.

If you are enrolling in an aerobics class, it is a good idea to check around for an instructor who plays music you like. Music can be either a major motivator or a major turnoff. Similarly, it is important that you find an instructor you feel comfortable with. Different instructors have different exercise styles as well as different attitudes. Check out a few classes before you commit yourself to one in particular. You will find this little bit of effort to be time well spent.

Be patient.

Don't expect to be able to master all of the moves immediately. Many of these classes require a fair degree of coordination. Be patient. Even the instructors didn't learn these moves overnight.

Start with the lowest step.

If you choose step aerobics, always start with the lowest possible step. It is also a good idea to forget about the arm movements and just concentrate on footwork until you get the hang of it.

Looking Back

This chapter began with the important function of helping you determine if exercise is safe for you. You were provided with established guidelines indicating whether or not a medical examination is necessary and were asked to complete the Personal Health Checklist. It is very important that you follow the advice in both of these sections. They will ensure your healthy and ongoing participation in physical activity. At this point, six specific exercises were described that have shown the most potential to improve mental health. In each instance, the advantages of the particular exercise, recommended equipment, proper technique, a sample program for beginners, and some final helpful hints were provided. By following the advice presented in this chapter, you have all of the information necessary to pick the physical activity that is best for you. The sample program will also get you started in a safe and progressive manner.

CHAPTER 6

STICKING WITH YOUR EXERCISE PROGRAM

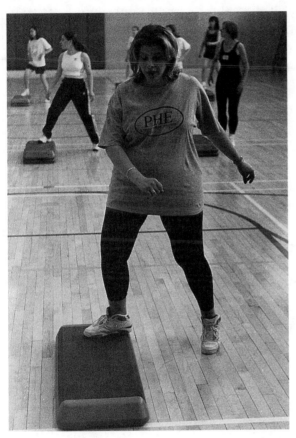

With few exceptions, most people have a choice as to whether or not they will stick with their exercise programs. Now that you have read about the positive effects of exercise on mental health and have been exposed to all the information you need about designing your own program, it is important for you to take one last step. Obviously, for exercise to have the desired benefits, it is necessary for you to stick with your program. Although this sounds easy in principle, the latest research paints an entirely different picture. In fact, it has now been estimated that over 50% of all people starting a structured exercise program will drop out within the first six months.

Given what we know about the physical and mental benefits of exercise, this 50% dropout rate presents us with a perplexing and difficult problem. How can we expect to improve our mental health through exercise if the

In this chapter, we will
- ✓ examine reasons why people continue exercising.
- ✓ examine reasons why people drop out.
- ✓ provide you with specific behavioral tools to help you stick with your program.

odds are poor that we will be able to stick with our programs? Fortunately, there are several workable solutions to this dropout problem. Some of them can be relatively simple. Consider the following example.

Brent's Buddy

Brent had finally convinced himself that it was time to get some exercise. He was especially attracted to the idea of weight training — an activity that would improve his conditioning and make him look better. After checking out a variety of fitness clubs, Brent finally decided on the one that was closest to his house. He remembered hearing that having exercise facilities that are close makes it easier to stick with the program. For the first month, Brent managed to work out three times per week, although it became increasingly tougher to motivate himself to exercise. He started missing more and more sessions until he finally quit going altogether. Fortunately, a few weeks later, in a conversation with a long-time friend, Brent talked about his new membership at the fitness club and how he had dropped out in a little over a month. Brent was surprised when his buddy told him that he also had been meaning to get involved in a fitness program. After a good discussion of the benefits of exercise, the two friends decided that they would work out together. On the designated exercise nights, they would take turns driving to the club. Each also agreed to serve as the other's "conscience" on days one of them didn't feel up to going. To the surprise of both, this worked great. After six months, both partners were still involved in regular weight training. Brent summed up their progress best when he said, "Although I know I could still talk myself out of exercising, I just can't bring myself to let my buddy down."

After reading this chapter and following a few simple principles, there is no reason you have to become another dropout statistic. Before examining these strategies in detail, let's take a moment to consider the reasons that determine whether or not a person will stick with an exercise program.

What Factors Predict Exercise Adherence?

To answer this question, a large study[1] was conducted in the United States. In this investigation, 1400 adults were questioned in terms of their health, jobs, lifestyles, beliefs, and overall psychological makeup. One year later, all of this information was compared to actual exercise behavior. As a result of these comparisons, several predictors of both exercise adherence and dropping out were determined. These results are summarized below.

FACTORS PREDICTING ADHERENCE
Self-motivation
Behavioral and coping skills
Support of spouse
Available time
Easy access to exercise facilities
Belief in own good health
High risk for heart disease

FACTORS PREDICTING DROPOUT
Blue-collar status
Overweight or obesity
Discomfort during exercise
Smoking

When you look at this list, you will see that some of these factors are more within your control than others are. For example, the amount of time you have available for exercise may be minimal because of job and family responsibilities. Similarly, your access to exercise facilities is fixed by where you live. Along the same lines, your actual vocation is something that is not readily changed in today's job market. Factors such as these are usually beyond your immediate control. Even so, later in this chapter you will be provided with several hints that will help you overcome these and other obstacles.

For the most part, what we want to do is focus on those factors that we can do something about. A sincere effort to quit smoking and to lose those extra pounds will go a long way in preventing you from becoming an exercise dropout. After that, it comes down to the two factors, self-motivation and behavioral and coping skills, that fall within your direct control. In reality, these two factors can be lumped together, since self-motivation is to a large extent determined by our behavioral and coping skills. In other words, if we use the correct behavioral techniques, this in turn will lead to greater self-motivation. For this reason, the remainder of this chapter will show you how to put these behavioral principles to work for you.

What Exactly Are Behavioral and Coping Skills?

When we talk about behavioral and coping skills, we are really referring to what are technically called behavior-change strategies. These change strategies, or "intervention techniques," have been developed over the years by research psychologists. They have proven to be effective for changing a wide range of behaviors, including smoking, drinking, studying, poor conduct, dieting, and even sexual problems.

Over the past several years, these same principles have been found effective for helping people stick with their exercise programs. In fact, in a recent study performed by this author,[2] 31 specific experiments were reviewed that attempted to change exercise behavior by means of behavioral strategies. The most important finding from this research is that 26 out of 31 (84%) studies reported improved exercise adherence. A second important finding was that all behavioral change strategies appeared equally effective.

These observations represent an amazing discovery. They suggest that using behavioral-change strategies is the single best way to keep a person involved in an exercise program and that the choice of intervention strategies can be largely a matter of personal taste.

Although there appears to be a good deal of room for personal choice of strategies, the four interventions that are used most often include the decision balance sheet, a formal contract, relapse-prevention training, and self-recording. For this reason, each of these strategies will now be examined in detail. Make sure that you complete each of the following exercises. If you do, the chances are excellent that you will have no trouble sticking with your exercise program.

Using the Decision Balance Sheet

The idea behind the decision balance sheet may not be entirely new to you. Oftentimes, when we have to make a decision of some kind, we try to jot down the "pros" and "cons" of each alternative. This helps us *weigh* our choices and come up with the correct answer. This is exactly what we do with the Exercise Decision Balance Sheet.

You will notice that the following worksheet is divided into two columns. On the left-hand side, you will notice the heading *Benefits/Advantages*. Under this heading, write down all of the benefits or advantages that you think would result from your participation in an exercise program. These can include physical, psychological, or even social benefits. The key here is to be thorough; the more inclusive your list, the more effective it will be.

Repeat this procedure under the *Costs/Disadvantages* heading. What problems, inconveniences, or costs do you foresee? Once again, be as thorough as possible.

EXERCISE DECISION BALANCE SHEET	
Benefits (Advantages)	Costs (Disadvantages)

If you have done a thorough job, you will probably notice that the list that you have made in your left-hand column is longer than the one in your right-hand one. This just confirms that starting an exercise program is the right decision for you.

Writing Up an Exercise Contract

An exercise contract is no different from any other type of contract. It commits you to a particular course of action. Most people have had experience with formal contracts of one kind or another. For example, it is usually necessary to sign a contract once you have been offered a job. Similarly, when you purchase a car, a formal sales contract is drawn up between you and the car company. The same situation applies when you purchase a house or condominium. In all of these cases, you are required to sign a specific contract.

The main idea behind these contracts is to set forth all of the conditions that must be met in order for the transaction to be considered completed. Once you have entered into such an agreement by means of your signature, it becomes difficult to break the contract. This same idea is at work with the Exercise Contract. By publicly committing yourself to the contract in the presence of a witness (who also signs the contract), you are making a strong statement in terms of your seriousness. So take a few minutes and fill out the following form. This will go a long way in helping you stick with your program.

EXERCISE CONTRACT

I,_____ , do hereby agree to perform the
following exercise(s) _____
_____ a
minimum of _____ times per week for a total of _____ weeks. Each exercise session will last a total of _____ minutes.

If I accomplish this goal, and abide by all of the conditions set forth
above, I will reward myself/be rewarded in the following manner:

_____
_____

If I fail to complete this contract by not performing all of the conditions stated herein, my punishment will be the following:

_____
_____
_____
_____

_____   _____
Participant Signature   Date

_____   _____
Witness Signature   Date

Now that you have publicly committed yourself to an exercise program,
it is important to anticipate some of the roadblocks that you may encounter
along the way. By developing a plan to deal with these possible setbacks, you
will be in a better position to stick with your program.

Using a Relapse-Prevention Training Worksheet

The main idea behind this behavioral technique is to get you thinking
about situations that may develop that will prevent you from completing your
workout on any given day. Although this sounds like negative thinking, it is
just the opposite. It requires you to develop a realistic view of everyday factors that have the potential to derail your exercise plans. The next step in the
process is to form an alternate strategy, or coping response, that will allow
you to get around the roadblock.

For example, let's say that you have decided to start a walking program.
You feel that Monday, Wednesday, and Friday evenings after supper would

be the best time for exercising. Your exercise goal, then, is to walk on these particular nights. You would write this goal in the left-hand column on the following worksheet. Now you ask yourself, "What could prevent me from accomplishing my goal?" One sample answer would be a heavy rainfall on one of your exercise nights. Another possibility would be a friend's coming over for a visit. Each of these situations presents a possible roadblock for your exercise program. You would write these possibilities down in the middle column of the following worksheet.

Your next task is to have a backup plan, or coping response, that will put you back on track. In the heavy rain example, a suitable coping response would be a "mall walk." Another possible solution would be to substitute another exercise night. You would write these, and any other solutions you can think of, in the right-hand column of the worksheet.

If you give this technique some serious thought, you will be able to develop coping responses for most of the potential roadblocks that may arise over the next several weeks. So take some time, and try to make your Relapse-Prevention Worksheet as thorough as possible. By putting in the effort now, your chances of completing your exercise program will be greatly improved. Remember, forewarned is forearmed.

RELAPSE-PREVENTION WORKSHEET

Exercise Goal	Possible Roadblock	Coping Response

Now that you are armed with a good plan for dealing with situations that might sidetrack you from your exercise goals, it is time to start your program.

The next technique we will be looking at has great potential for keeping you involved.

Self-Recording Your Exercise

One of the best strategies for sticking with your exercise program is simple. It requires you to record, or write down, the exercises that you complete on any given day. This will provide a written record of your exercise program. You can also record such items as the weather, your mood before and after exercise, and any other piece of information that is important to you on that day.

To help you with this process, chapter 7 provides you with your own exercise diary. This will allow you to record your exercise efforts for a 12-week period. By the time you complete this diary, exercise will have already become a regular part of your lifestyle.

Now that you have all the information that you need to put these four behavioral techniques to work for you, read through the following section. It will provide other behavior change hints. Don't think that you have to perform them all. This is where your personal choice comes in. Simply read through the following hints and pick one or two that you think would work best for you. Then give them a try. Feel free to experiment with different hints until you find the ones that are most effective for you.

Some Final Helpful Hints

Choose your activity carefully, but choose.

You will find it easier to stick with your program if you have chosen the type of exercise yourself. Joining programs where you have no say in choosing the activities often leads to dropping out. Also, whenever possible, select an exercise that is convenient to perform and readily accessible. The farther you have to travel to exercise and the more complicated the activity, the easier it is to skip the day's session.

Seek social support.

Support from significant others, such as your spouse, another family member, or a close friend has been shown to be every bit as important as the exerciser's attitude itself. All of us need a "pat on the back" from time to time to help us persist with our efforts. If you have this support already, your chances of sticking with your program are greatly improved. If you don't currently have this support, don't be shy — seek it out. The results will be well worth your efforts.

Don't feel you have to do it alone.

Many exercisers find it beneficial to work out in a small group. You will be less likely to skip exercise sessions because you would be letting your partners down. If small group exercise is not for you, try the "buddy system." Find a friend with similar exercise goals; then determine suitable times for participation. Once again, you will be more likely to stick with your program because you don't want to skip out on your exercise partner.

Don't overdo it.

Try to exercise at a mild- or moderate-intensity level. The majority of people do not remain in exercise programs when the activity is too vigorous. To determine the proper workout intensity for you, use the "talk-test." When exercising, you should be able to comfortably carry on a conversation with your exercise partner. If you find you are becoming too tired to talk comfortably, you are exercising too hard. Slow down, take it easy, and enjoy yourself.

Reward yourself early.

If you have met your first week's exercise goals, make sure you reward yourself. Take in a movie, or treat yourself to that new paperback novel that you have been wanting. After your first successful month of exercise, reward yourself again. Do something nice for yourself, like going out to dinner with your spouse or a good friend. Make it a special celebration. You deserve it.

Consider using stimulus cuing.

Experiment with techniques such as placing your walking shoes just inside the front door or keeping your workout clothes in the car or at the office. They will be the first thing you see when you come home from work or shopping. This will "cue" you to go for that walk. Morning exercisers may find it helpful to hang their sweatsuit on the bedpost so it is the first item they see when they wake up. This serves as a powerful reminder to get in that exercise session.

Effective goal setting has been found helpful.

People who set appropriate goals have an easier time sticking with their exercise programs. To be effective, your goals must be observable, measurable, and achievable. In other words, it is important that you be able to "see" the successful completion of a goal. Similarly, your goal must be a realistic one. If it is too difficult to achieve, this can be demoralizing. On the other hand, goals that are too easy are not motivating. So take care to set goals that are challenging but well within your reach. You can always make goal adjustments later if you find your initial goals are too easy to accomplish. Another effective goal-setting technique involves being specific. It is much better to say you are going to exercise Monday, Wednesday, and Friday at 11:00 A.M. than it is to merely say three times per week. The latter case gives you too much opportunity to put off your exercise session.

Use a favorite activity to reward your exercise efforts.

If there is a particular activity you like to do each day, like reading or watching TV, don't allow yourself to perform that activity on exercise days until *after* your workout. With this technique, one of your preferred pastimes actually becomes a reward for completing an exercise session.

Learn to prevent unwanted distractions.

Try to identify, then avoid, those situations that tend to cause you to skip your exercise sessions. Sample distractions might be television, shopping sprees, or socializing. While all of these activities are enjoyable on their own, it is important to keep track of those events that sidetrack you, then try to avoid them completely on exercise days. There will be many more opportunities for all of these activities during the rest of the week.

Use some variety in your workouts.

Learn to avoid boredom by substituting different exercises from time to time. If you have selected a jogging program, don't hesitate to substitute a walk or a swim occasionally. Adding some variety will spice up your exercise program and break the monotony of performing the same activity all the time.

Learn to dissociate from your exercise.

Most people report that exercising is easier when they think about unrelated things, such as a movie, a friend, or other pleasant experiences. Other people find it helpful to listen to music on a Walkman. So let your mind wander a bit, and don't dwell exclusively on the exercise itself. Focusing on the physical activity serves to remind us of feelings of fatigue and makes the effort more of a chore.

Use self-talk to help yourself stick with the activity.

Don't be embarrassed to use self-statements such as, "Way to go — I'm really sticking with my program," or, "Today, I'm going to have a great workout." Statements such as these have been found to be effective in making us feel better about ourselves and helping us stick with our programs. You may feel more comfortable, and you will certainly draw fewer stares, if you make these self-statements silently, and do not say them out loud.

Looking Back

Chapter 6 might just be the most important part of this book. Up to this point, you have been provided with all the information needed to choose an exercise that will improve your mental health. While all of this information is valuable, it will ultimately be of little use if you are unable to stick with your program. For this reason, you were provided with a series of behavioral and coping skills that will keep you involved on a long-term basis. The Exercise Decision Balance Sheet and the Exercise Contract will both help get you started. The Relapse-Prevention Worksheet and the variety of other behavioral hints presented will help you maintain your involvement. As a final, and very important adherence tool, a Personal Exercise Diary (chapter 7) is provided: here you are encouraged to record your exercise habits and daily mood. So turn to the next chapter and start recording your progress. You will find this to be an excellent motivator to stick with your program.

Note

1 Sallis, J.F., Haskell, W.L., Fortmann, S.P., Vranizan, K.M., Taylor, C.B., & Solomon, D.S. (1986). Predictors of adoption and maintenance of physical activity in a community sample. *Preventive Medicine, 15,* 331–341.

2 Leith, L.M., & Taylor, A.H. (1992). Behavior modification and exercise adherence: A literature review. *Journal of Sport Behavior, 16,* 1–15.

PERSONAL EXERCISE DIARY

In chapter 5, you read how self-recording your exercise is a proven technique to help you stick with your program. For this reason, chapter 7 provides you with your exercise diary. The diary is provided for 12 weeks, since this is the amount of time needed to notice improvements in self-concept. Reducing depression or anxiety requires slightly less time.

Twelve weeks is also about the length of time you need to persist with an exercise program before it becomes a way of life, with reduced chances of dropping out of your program. So make a deal with yourself to stick with your program until you have completed all 12 weeks. At that time, you will likely want to continue indefinitely. The tools provided in the previous chapter will help you succeed.

You will find it beneficial to record the following items in your diary:

- your weekly exercise goals
- the date of your exercise
- the type of exercise you perform
- how long you exercised and how hard it was for you
- your mood that day
- any other thoughts that are important to you
- an overview of your week's efforts
- your overall mood for the week

WEEK 1

THIS WEEK'S EXERCISE GOALS: _____

_____

_____

MONDAY: _____

EXERCISE PERFORMED TODAY: _____

_____

OTHER COMMENTS/TODAY'S MOOD: _____

_____

_____

TUESDAY: _____

EXERCISE PERFORMED TODAY: _____

_____

OTHER COMMENTS/TODAY'S MOOD: _____

_____

_____

WEDNESDAY: _____

EXERCISE PERFORMED TODAY: _____

_____

OTHER COMMENTS/TODAY'S MOOD: _____

_____

_____

THURSDAY: _____

EXERCISE PERFORMED TODAY: _____

_____

OTHER COMMENTS/TODAY'S MOOD: _____

_____

_____

FRIDAY: _____

EXERCISE PERFORMED TODAY: _____

_____

OTHER COMMENTS/TODAY'S MOOD: _____

_____

_____

SATURDAY: _____

EXERCISE PERFORMED TODAY: _____

_____

OTHER COMMENTS/TODAY'S MOOD: _____

_____

_____

SUNDAY: _____

EXERCISE PERFORMED TODAY: _____

_____

OTHER COMMENTS/TODAY'S MOOD: _____

_____

_____

MY WEEK IN REVIEW: _____

_____

_____

_____

_____

_____

HOW WAS MY MOOD THIS WEEK?

( )   ( )   ( )   ( )   ( )

Terrible   Poor   So-So   Good   Great

WEEK 2

THIS WEEK'S EXERCISE GOALS: _____

_____

_____

MONDAY: _____

EXERCISE PERFORMED TODAY: _____

_____

OTHER COMMENTS/TODAY'S MOOD: _____

_____

_____

TUESDAY: _____

EXERCISE PERFORMED TODAY: _____

_____

OTHER COMMENTS/TODAY'S MOOD: _____

_____

_____

WEDNESDAY: _____

EXERCISE PERFORMED TODAY: _____

_____

OTHER COMMENTS/TODAY'S MOOD: _____

_____

_____

THURSDAY: _____

EXERCISE PERFORMED TODAY: _____

_____

OTHER COMMENTS/TODAY'S MOOD: _____

_____

_____

FRIDAY: _____

EXERCISE PERFORMED TODAY: _____

_____

OTHER COMMENTS/TODAY'S MOOD: _____

_____

_____

SATURDAY: _____

EXERCISE PERFORMED TODAY: _____

_____

OTHER COMMENTS/TODAY'S MOOD: _____

_____

_____

SUNDAY: _____

EXERCISE PERFORMED TODAY: _____

_____

OTHER COMMENTS/TODAY'S MOOD: _____

_____

_____

MY WEEK IN REVIEW: _____

_____

_____

_____

_____

_____

HOW WAS MY MOOD THIS WEEK?

( )   ( )   ( )   ( )   ( )
Terrible   Poor   So-So   Good   Great

WEEK 3

THIS WEEK'S EXERCISE GOALS: _____

_____

_____

MONDAY: _____

EXERCISE PERFORMED TODAY: _____

_____

OTHER COMMENTS/TODAY'S MOOD: _____

_____

_____

TUESDAY: _____

EXERCISE PERFORMED TODAY: _____

_____

OTHER COMMENTS/TODAY'S MOOD: _____

_____

_____

WEDNESDAY: _____

EXERCISE PERFORMED TODAY: _____

_____

OTHER COMMENTS/TODAY'S MOOD: _____

_____

_____

THURSDAY: _____

EXERCISE PERFORMED TODAY: _____

_____

OTHER COMMENTS/TODAY'S MOOD: _____

_____

_____

FRIDAY: _____

EXERCISE PERFORMED TODAY: _____

_____

OTHER COMMENTS/TODAY'S MOOD: _____

_____

_____

SATURDAY: _____

EXERCISE PERFORMED TODAY: _____

_____

OTHER COMMENTS/TODAY'S MOOD: _____

_____

_____

SUNDAY: _____

EXERCISE PERFORMED TODAY: _____

_____

OTHER COMMENTS/TODAY'S MOOD: _____

_____

_____

MY WEEK IN REVIEW: _____

_____

_____

_____

_____

_____

HOW WAS MY MOOD THIS WEEK?

( )   ( )   ( )   ( )   ( )

Terrible   Poor   So-So   Good   Great

WEEK 4

THIS WEEK'S EXERCISE GOALS: _____

_____

_____

MONDAY: _____

EXERCISE PERFORMED TODAY: _____

_____

OTHER COMMENTS/TODAY'S MOOD: _____

_____

_____

TUESDAY: _____

EXERCISE PERFORMED TODAY: _____

_____

OTHER COMMENTS/TODAY'S MOOD: _____

_____

_____

WEDNESDAY: _____

EXERCISE PERFORMED TODAY: _____

_____

OTHER COMMENTS/TODAY'S MOOD: _____

_____

_____

THURSDAY: _____

EXERCISE PERFORMED TODAY: _____

_____

OTHER COMMENTS/TODAY'S MOOD: _____

_____

_____

FRIDAY: _____

EXERCISE PERFORMED TODAY: _____

_____

OTHER COMMENTS/TODAY'S MOOD: _____

_____

_____

SATURDAY: _____

EXERCISE PERFORMED TODAY: _____

_____

OTHER COMMENTS/TODAY'S MOOD: _____

_____

_____

SUNDAY: _____

EXERCISE PERFORMED TODAY: _____

_____

OTHER COMMENTS/TODAY'S MOOD: _____

_____

_____

MY WEEK IN REVIEW: _____

_____

_____

_____

_____

HOW WAS MY MOOD THIS WEEK?

( )   ( )   ( )   ( )   ( )

Terrible   Poor   So-So   Good   Great

WEEK 5

THIS WEEK'S EXERCISE GOALS: _____

_____

_____

MONDAY: _____

EXERCISE PERFORMED TODAY: _____

_____

OTHER COMMENTS/TODAY'S MOOD: _____

_____

_____

TUESDAY: _____

EXERCISE PERFORMED TODAY: _____

_____

OTHER COMMENTS/TODAY'S MOOD: _____

_____

_____

WEDNESDAY: _____

EXERCISE PERFORMED TODAY: _____

_____

OTHER COMMENTS/TODAY'S MOOD: _____

_____

_____

THURSDAY: _____

EXERCISE PERFORMED TODAY: _____

_____

OTHER COMMENTS/TODAY'S MOOD: _____

_____

_____

FRIDAY: _____

EXERCISE PERFORMED TODAY: _____

_____

OTHER COMMENTS/TODAY'S MOOD: _____

_____

_____

SATURDAY: _____

EXERCISE PERFORMED TODAY: _____

_____

OTHER COMMENTS/TODAY'S MOOD: _____

_____

_____

SUNDAY: _____

EXERCISE PERFORMED TODAY: _____

_____

OTHER COMMENTS/TODAY'S MOOD: _____

_____

_____

MY WEEK IN REVIEW: _____

_____

_____

_____

_____

_____

HOW WAS MY MOOD THIS WEEK?

( )   ( )   ( )   ( )   ( )

Terrible   Poor   So-So   Good   Great

WEEK 6

THIS WEEK'S EXERCISE GOALS: _____

_____

_____

MONDAY: _____

EXERCISE PERFORMED TODAY: _____

_____

OTHER COMMENTS/TODAY'S MOOD: _____

_____

_____

TUESDAY: _____

EXERCISE PERFORMED TODAY: _____

_____

OTHER COMMENTS/TODAY'S MOOD: _____

_____

_____

WEDNESDAY: _____

EXERCISE PERFORMED TODAY: _____

_____

OTHER COMMENTS/TODAY'S MOOD: _____

_____

_____

THURSDAY: _____

EXERCISE PERFORMED TODAY: _____

_____

OTHER COMMENTS/TODAY'S MOOD: _____

_____

_____

FRIDAY: _____

EXERCISE PERFORMED TODAY: _____

_____

OTHER COMMENTS/TODAY'S MOOD: _____

_____

_____

SATURDAY: _____

EXERCISE PERFORMED TODAY: _____

_____

OTHER COMMENTS/TODAY'S MOOD: _____

_____

_____

SUNDAY: _____

EXERCISE PERFORMED TODAY: _____

_____

OTHER COMMENTS/TODAY'S MOOD: _____

_____

_____

MY WEEK IN REVIEW: _____

_____

_____

_____

_____

_____

HOW WAS MY MOOD THIS WEEK?

( )	( )	( )	( )	( )
Terrible	Poor	So-So	Good	Great

WEEK 7

THIS WEEK'S EXERCISE GOALS: _____

_____

MONDAY: _____

EXERCISE PERFORMED TODAY: _____

OTHER COMMENTS/TODAY'S MOOD: _____

_____

TUESDAY: _____

EXERCISE PERFORMED TODAY: _____

OTHER COMMENTS/TODAY'S MOOD: _____

_____

WEDNESDAY: _____

EXERCISE PERFORMED TODAY: _____

OTHER COMMENTS/TODAY'S MOOD: _____

_____

THURSDAY: _____

EXERCISE PERFORMED TODAY: _____

OTHER COMMENTS/TODAY'S MOOD: _____

_____

FRIDAY: _____

EXERCISE PERFORMED TODAY: _____

_____

OTHER COMMENTS/TODAY'S MOOD: _____

_____

_____

SATURDAY: _____

EXERCISE PERFORMED TODAY: _____

_____

OTHER COMMENTS/TODAY'S MOOD: _____

_____

_____

SUNDAY: _____

EXERCISE PERFORMED TODAY: _____

_____

OTHER COMMENTS/TODAY'S MOOD: _____

_____

_____

MY WEEK IN REVIEW: _____

_____

_____

_____

_____

_____

HOW WAS MY MOOD THIS WEEK?

( )   ( )   ( )   ( )   ( )

Terrible   Poor   So-So   Good   Great

WEEK 8

THIS WEEK'S EXERCISE GOALS: _____

_____

_____

MONDAY: _____

EXERCISE PERFORMED TODAY: _____

_____

OTHER COMMENTS/TODAY'S MOOD: _____

_____

_____

TUESDAY: _____

EXERCISE PERFORMED TODAY: _____

_____

OTHER COMMENTS/TODAY'S MOOD: _____

_____

_____

WEDNESDAY: _____

EXERCISE PERFORMED TODAY: _____

_____

OTHER COMMENTS/TODAY'S MOOD: _____

_____

_____

THURSDAY: _____

EXERCISE PERFORMED TODAY: _____

_____

OTHER COMMENTS/TODAY'S MOOD: _____

_____

_____

FRIDAY: _____

EXERCISE PERFORMED TODAY: _____

_____

OTHER COMMENTS/TODAY'S MOOD: _____

_____

_____

SATURDAY: _____

EXERCISE PERFORMED TODAY: _____

_____

OTHER COMMENTS/TODAY'S MOOD: _____

_____

_____

SUNDAY: _____

EXERCISE PERFORMED TODAY: _____

_____

OTHER COMMENTS/TODAY'S MOOD: _____

_____

_____

MY WEEK IN REVIEW: _____

_____

_____

_____

_____

_____

HOW WAS MY MOOD THIS WEEK?

( )	( )	( )	( )	( )
Terrible	Poor	So-So	Good	Great

WEEK 9

THIS WEEK'S EXERCISE GOALS: _____

_____

_____

MONDAY: _____

EXERCISE PERFORMED TODAY: _____

_____

OTHER COMMENTS/TODAY'S MOOD: _____

_____

_____

TUESDAY: _____

EXERCISE PERFORMED TODAY: _____

_____

OTHER COMMENTS/TODAY'S MOOD: _____

_____

_____

WEDNESDAY: _____

EXERCISE PERFORMED TODAY: _____

_____

OTHER COMMENTS/TODAY'S MOOD: _____

_____

_____

THURSDAY: _____

EXERCISE PERFORMED TODAY: _____

_____

OTHER COMMENTS/TODAY'S MOOD: _____

_____

_____

FRIDAY: _____

EXERCISE PERFORMED TODAY: _____

_____

OTHER COMMENTS/TODAY'S MOOD: _____

_____

_____

SATURDAY: _____

EXERCISE PERFORMED TODAY: _____

_____

OTHER COMMENTS/TODAY'S MOOD: _____

_____

_____

SUNDAY: _____

EXERCISE PERFORMED TODAY: _____

_____

OTHER COMMENTS/TODAY'S MOOD: _____

_____

_____

MY WEEK IN REVIEW: _____

_____

_____

_____

_____

_____

HOW WAS MY MOOD THIS WEEK?

( )   ( )   ( )   ( )   ( )

Terrible   Poor   So-So   Good   Great

WEEK 10

THIS WEEK'S EXERCISE GOALS: _____

_____

_____

MONDAY: _____

EXERCISE PERFORMED TODAY: _____

_____

OTHER COMMENTS/TODAY'S MOOD: _____

_____

_____

TUESDAY: _____

EXERCISE PERFORMED TODAY: _____

_____

OTHER COMMENTS/TODAY'S MOOD: _____

_____

_____

WEDNESDAY: _____

EXERCISE PERFORMED TODAY: _____

_____

OTHER COMMENTS/TODAY'S MOOD: _____

_____

_____

THURSDAY: _____

EXERCISE PERFORMED TODAY: _____

_____

OTHER COMMENTS/TODAY'S MOOD: _____

_____

_____

FRIDAY: _____

EXERCISE PERFORMED TODAY: _____

_____

OTHER COMMENTS/TODAY'S MOOD: _____

_____

_____

SATURDAY: _____

EXERCISE PERFORMED TODAY: _____

_____

OTHER COMMENTS/TODAY'S MOOD: _____

_____

_____

SUNDAY: _____

EXERCISE PERFORMED TODAY: _____

_____

OTHER COMMENTS/TODAY'S MOOD: _____

_____

_____

MY WEEK IN REVIEW: _____

_____

_____

_____

_____

HOW WAS MY MOOD THIS WEEK?

( )   ( )   ( )   ( )   ( )
Terrible   Poor   So-So   Good   Great

WEEK 11

THIS WEEK'S EXERCISE GOALS: _____
_____
_____

MONDAY: _____

EXERCISE PERFORMED TODAY: _____
_____

OTHER COMMENTS/TODAY'S MOOD: _____
_____
_____

TUESDAY: _____

EXERCISE PERFORMED TODAY: _____
_____

OTHER COMMENTS/TODAY'S MOOD: _____
_____
_____

WEDNESDAY: _____

EXERCISE PERFORMED TODAY: _____
_____

OTHER COMMENTS/TODAY'S MOOD: _____
_____
_____

THURSDAY: _____

EXERCISE PERFORMED TODAY: _____
_____

OTHER COMMENTS/TODAY'S MOOD: _____
_____
_____

FRIDAY: _____

EXERCISE PERFORMED TODAY: _____

_____

OTHER COMMENTS/TODAY'S MOOD: _____

_____

_____

SATURDAY: _____

EXERCISE PERFORMED TODAY: _____

_____

OTHER COMMENTS/TODAY'S MOOD: _____

_____

_____

SUNDAY: _____

EXERCISE PERFORMED TODAY: _____

_____

OTHER COMMENTS/TODAY'S MOOD: _____

_____

_____

MY WEEK IN REVIEW: _____

_____

_____

_____

_____

_____

HOW WAS MY MOOD THIS WEEK?

Terrible	Poor	So-So	Good	Great
( )	( )	( )	( )	( )

WEEK 12

THIS WEEK'S EXERCISE GOALS: _____

_____

_____

MONDAY: _____

EXERCISE PERFORMED TODAY: _____

_____

OTHER COMMENTS/TODAY'S MOOD: _____

_____

_____

TUESDAY: _____

EXERCISE PERFORMED TODAY: _____

_____

OTHER COMMENTS/TODAY'S MOOD: _____

_____

_____

WEDNESDAY: _____

EXERCISE PERFORMED TODAY: _____

_____

OTHER COMMENTS/TODAY'S MOOD: _____

_____

_____

THURSDAY: _____

EXERCISE PERFORMED TODAY: _____

_____

OTHER COMMENTS/TODAY'S MOOD: _____

_____

_____

FRIDAY: _____

EXERCISE PERFORMED TODAY: _____

_____

OTHER COMMENTS/TODAY'S MOOD: _____

_____

_____

SATURDAY: _____

EXERCISE PERFORMED TODAY: _____

_____

OTHER COMMENTS/TODAY'S MOOD: _____

_____

_____

SUNDAY: _____

EXERCISE PERFORMED TODAY: _____

_____

OTHER COMMENTS/TODAY'S MOOD: _____

_____

_____

MY WEEK IN REVIEW: _____

_____

_____

_____

_____

_____

HOW WAS MY MOOD THIS WEEK?

( )   ( )   ( )   ( )   ( )
Terrible   Poor   So-So   Good   Great

Suggested Readings

Anderson, W. (1997). *The confidence course*. New York: HarperCollins.
This book includes 20 interactive lessons that will teach you how to overcome crippling self-doubt.

Burke, E.R. (1996). *Complete home fitness handbook*. Champaign, IL: Human Kinetics.
This book tells you how you can get in great shape without leaving home. It discusses machine weights, stationary cycles, stair climbers, treadmills, and ski machines.

Burns, D.D. (1989). *The feeling good handbook*. New York: Penguin Books.
This book provides step-by-step exercises that help you fight depression without the use of medication.

Burns, D.D. (1992). *Feeling good : The new mood therapy*. New York: Penguin Books.
This books shows you how to overcome cognitive distortions that affect the way you view yourself.

Copeland, M.E. (1992). *The depression workbook*. Oakland, CA: New Harbinger Publications, Inc.
Through a series of personal awareness exercises, this book helps you track and control your moods, thereby taking responsibility for your own wellness.

Eliot, R.S. (1994). *From stress to strength*. New York: Bantam Books.
This book utilizes a 40-point Quality of Life Index that allows you to assess your risks and transform stressful situations into productive ones.

Powell, T. (1997). *Free yourself from harmful stress*. Montreal: Reader's Digest.
This book helps you recognize the physical and emotional symptoms of stress and its sources, then provides the skills for managing that stress in the future.

Schlosberg, S., & Neporent, L. (1996). *Fitness for dummies*. Foster City, CA: IDG Books Worldwide, Inc.
This book is an excellent guide for choosing a health club, buying exercise equipment, designing your workout, and more.

Index